Reversing the Tide

Priorities for HIV/AIDS Prevention in Central Asia

Joana Godinho
Adrian Renton
Viatcheslav Vinogradov
Thomas Novotny
Mary-Jane Rivers
George Gotsadze
Mario Bravo

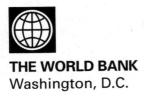

THE WORLD BANK
Washington, D.C.

World Bank Working Papers are published to communicate the results of the Bank's work to the development community with the least possible delay. The manuscript of this paper therefore has not been prepared in accordance with the procedures appropriate to formally-edited texts. Some sources cited in this paper may be informal documents that are not readily available.

The findings, interpretations, and conclusions expressed herein are those of the author(s) and do not necessarily reflect the views of the International Bank for Reconstruction and Development/The World Bank and its affiliated organizations, or those of the Executive Directors of The World Bank or the governments they represent.

The World Bank does not guarantee the accuracy of the data included in this work. The boundaries, colors, denominations, and other information shown on any map in this work do not imply and judgment on the part of The World Bank of the legal status of any territory or the endorsement or acceptance of such boundaries.

The material in this publication is copyrighted. Copying and/or transmitting portions or all of this work without permission may be a violation of applicable law. The International Bank for Reconstruction and Development/The World Bank encourages dissemination of its work and will normally grant permission promptly to reproduce portions of the work.

For permission to photocopy or reprint any part of this work, please send a request with complete information to the Copyright Clearance Center, Inc., 222 Rosewood Drive, Danvers, MA 01923, USA, Tel: 978-750-8400, Fax: 978-750-4470, www.copyright.com.

All other queries on rights and licenses, including subsidiary rights, should be addressed to the Office of the Publisher, The World Bank, 1818 H Street NW, Washington, DC 20433, USA, Fax: 202-522-2422, email: pubrights@worldbank.org.

ISBN-10: 0-8213-6230-5   ISBN-13: 978-0-8213-6230-3
eISBN: 0-8213-6231-3
ISSN: 1726-5878   DOI: 10.1596/978-0-8213-6230-3

Joana Godinho is a Senior Health Specialist at the Human Development Department of the World Bank. Adrian Renton is a Reader in Social Medicine, Department of Social Science and Medicine, Imperial College School of Medicine. Viatcheslav Vinogradov is a Professor at the Center for Economic Research & Graduate Education, Czech Economic Institute. Thomas Novotny is the Director of International Educational Programs, Institute for Global Health, School of Medicine at the University of California, San Francisco. Mary-Jane Rivers is a Social Scientist at Delta Networks, New Zealand. George Gotsadze is the Director of the Curatio International Foundation. Mario Bravo is a Senior Communication Specialist, The World Bank.

Library of Congress Cataloging-in-Publication Data has been requested.

Contents

LIST OF BOXES

UNNUMBERED BOXES

Dedication

This study is dedicated to Rudik Adamian, the late UNAIDS Regional Coordinator, who significantly contributed for early prevention of HIV/AIDS in Central Asia

Acknowledgments

This study was prepared by a team led by Joana Godinho. Background papers were prepared by the following co-authors: Epidemiological Overview of HIV/AIDS and STIs in Central Asia by Adrian Renton; The Economic Consequences of HIV in Central Asia by Viatcheslav Vinogradov; Strategic and Regulatory Framework in Central Asia by Thomas Novotny; Stakeholder Analysis and Institutional Assessment by Mary-Jane Rivers and George Gotsadze; and the Communication Plan by Mario Bravo. Elina Manjieva assisted the preparation of the paper for publication.[1]

The team would like to acknowledge the contribution of James Cercone to the identification of key emerging issues on HIV/AIDS in Central Asia, Andrew Amato-Gauci and Nina Kerimi for their contribution to the stakeholder analysis and institutional assessment in Tajikistan and Turkmenistan respectively, and Dorothee Eckertz for preparing the tables on funding of HIV/AIDS Programs in Central Asia. In addition, Baktybek Zhumadil, Dinara Djoldosheva, Asel Sargaldakova, Natalia Turchina, Jamshed Khasanov, Janna Yunusova, Janna Yusupjanova, Dilnara Isamiddinova, and Gulnora Kamilova provided data and organized meetings with counterparts and other stakeholders in their respective countries: Kazakhstan, Kyrgyz Republic, Tajikistan, Turkmenistan, and Uzbekistan.

The study team is thankful to James Christopher Lovelace, Country Manager in the Kyrgyz Republic, and Armin Fidler, Sector Manager, for their comments and support; to the Study Peer Reviewers—Martha Ainsworth (OED) and Nina Schwalbe (OSI)—for their helpful insights; to Martin Hall, from the Imperial College in London, for his comments on the study of the potential economic impact of the epidemic; and to all other colleagues that have contributed with their helpful comments to the final report.

The study team is grateful to the Governments of Kazakhstan, Kyrgyz Republic, Tajikistan and Uzbekistan for their openness, which made this and other Central Asia AIDS and TB studies possible. The team is especially grateful to the Ministries of Health, Justice, Internal Affairs and Finances; AIDS Centers from Central Asian countries; as well as to all regional partners and NGOs that provided data and participated in meetings to discuss the main issues identified.

The World Bank		
Vice President	:	Shigeo Katsu
Country Director	:	Dennis de Tray
Sector Director	:	Charles Griffin
Sector Manager	:	Armin Fidler
Task Team Leader	:	Joana Godinho

1. Joana Godinho is a Senior Health Specialist at the Human Development Department of the World Bank. Adrian Renton is a Reader in Social Medicine, Department of Social Science and Medicine, Imperial College School of Medicine. Viatcheslav Vinogradov is a Professor at the Center for Economic Research & Graduate Education, Czech Economic Institute. Thomas Novotny is the Director of International Educational Programs, Institute for Global Health, School of Medicine at the University of California, San Francisco. Mary-Jane Rivers is a Social Scientist at Delta Networks, New Zealand. George Gotsadze is the Director of Curatio International Foundation, Georgia. Mario Bravo is a Senior Communications Officer at the External Department of the World Bank.

Acronyms and Abbreviations

AFEW	AIDS Foundation East-West
AIDS	Acquired Immune Deficiency Syndrome
ARV	Antiretroviral
CA	Central Asia
CAR	Central Asia Republics
CCM	Country Coordination Mechanism
CDC	Centers for Disease Control and Prevention
CSW	Commercial Sex Worker
DCA	Drug Control Agency
DFID	Department for International Development
DOTS	TB Directly Observed Therapy Short-Course
ECA	Europe and Central Asia
ECA/EXT	Europe and Central Asia, External Affairs
ECAVP	Europe and Central Asia, Office of the Vice President
ESCM	Electronic Surveillance Case-Based Management System
FM	Family Medicine
FSU	Former Soviet Union
FPG	Family Practice Group
GAR	Groups at Risk
GDF	Global Drug Facility
GFATM	Global Fund to Fight AIDS, TB & Malaria
GoK	Government of Kyrgyz Republic
GoT	Government of Tajikistan
GoU	Government of Uzbekistan
HFA	Health for All
HIV	Human Immunodeficiency Virus
HR	Harm Reduction
IA	Institutional Assessment
IDA	International Development Association
IDU	Injecting Drug User
IEC	Information, Education and Communication Campaign
IFRC	International Federation of Red Cross
IHRD	International Harm Reduction Network
IHRP	International Harm Reduction Program
IO	International Organizations
IOM	International Organization for Migration
IPPF	International Planned Parenthood Federation
IUATLD	International Union against Tuberculosis and Lung Disease
JICA	Japan International Cooperation Agency
KAP	Knowledge, Attitudes and Practices
KfW	German Development Bank (Kreditanstalt für Wiederaufbau)
MDGs	Millennium Development Goals

MDRTB	Multi-Drug Resistant Tuberculosis
MMR	Mass Miniature Radiography (fluorography)
MOH	Ministry of Health
MOIA	Ministry of Internal Affaires
MOJ	Ministry of Justice
MRT	Methadone Replacement therapy
MSF	Médecins Sans Frontières
MSM	Men who have sex with men
MTCT	Mother to Child Transmission of HIV/AIDS
NGO	Non Governmental Organizations
NTP	National Tuberculosis Program
OECD	Organization for Economic Cooperation and Development
OSI/Soros Foundation	Open Society Institute/Soros Foundation
PCN	Project Concept Note
PHC	Primary Health Care
PLWHA	People Living with HIV/AIDS
PRM	Participatory Resource Mapping
PSI	Population Services International
RAR	Rapid Assessment Response
RDU	Registered Drug User
RM	World Bank Resident Missions
SA	Stakeholder Analysis
SFK	Soros Foundation Kazakhstan
STI	Sexually Transmitted Infection
TB	Tuberculosis
TG	UN AIDS Thematic Group
TOR	Terms of Reference
UNAIDS	Joint United Nations Program on HIV/AIDS
UNDP	United Nations Development Program
UNFPA	United Nations Fund for Population Assistance
UNHCR	UN High Commission on Refugees
UNICEF	United Nations International Children's Fund
UNODC	UN Office for Drug Control and Crime Prevention
USAID	United States Agency for International Development
VCT	Voluntary Testing and Counseling
VDRL	Test for syphilis
WHO	World Health Organization

Executive Summary

This Study aims to identify strategies for ensuring early and effective intervention to control the AIDS epidemic in Central Asia at national and regional levels, considering priorities based on global evidence. It also aims to inform the Bank's policy dialogue and the operational work to control HIV/AIDS in Central Asia, and to strengthen the regional partnership between Governments, civil society, UN agencies, and multilateral and bilateral agencies to prevent HIV/AIDS and STIs.

Central Asia[2] has been confronting four overlapping epidemics—drug use, sexually transmitted infections (STIs), HIV/AIDS, and tuberculosis (TB). The drug use, HIV/AIDS, and STIs epidemics are mainly among young adults, while the TB epidemic affects adults in their more economically productive years. Although the number of reported cases of HIV in Central Asia is still very low, the growth rate of the epidemic—from about 500 cases in 2000 to over 12,000 in 2004—is a cause for serious concern.[3] Central Asia lies along the drug routes from Afghanistan to Russia and Western Europe, and it is estimated that it has half a million drug users, of which more than half inject drugs. The majority of users are men under 35, although drug use is increasing rapidly among women. However, HIV infection incidence and prevalence are estimated to be several times higher than reported figures. The lack of accuracy in reporting stems from the lack of proper diagnostic systems and the absence of an efficient surveillance system.

Current and future epidemic outbreaks of HIV throughout the region may continue to be driven by: a) the explosive growth in injecting drug and commercial sex work use; b) concurrent epidemics of sexually transmitted infections (STIs); c) economic and political migration; d) limited capacity of governments and civil society to implement effective preventive responses; and e) low levels of awareness of HIV and STIs and of knowledge about risk practices and protection. These conditions arise from economic decline since independence, as well as high volumes of illicit drug transit through the region and growth of local consumer markets for these drugs.

Therefore, the countries of Central Asia are highly vulnerable to an HIV/AIDS crisis over the next 20 years. Without concerted action, we may expect to see the rapid development over 4–5 years of an HIV epidemic concentrated among injecting drug users, followed by spread in the general population aged 15–30 years, with sexual transmission as the predominant mode. This would follow the pattern of the epidemic in other regional countries such as Russia, Ukraine and Moldova.

Governments, NGOs, and international partners in the field have taken initial steps to avoid a major HIV/AIDS epidemic in Central Asia. All countries with the exception of Turkmenistan have put in place coherent overarching policies and strategies to control HIV, which were prepared with assistance from UNAIDS; and have applied for grants from the Global Fund to Fight AIDS, TB, and Malaria (GFATM), which have been granted

---

2. Central Asia includes Kazakhstan, Kyrgyz Republic, Tajikistan, Turkmenistan and Uzbekistan.
3. The data were provided by the Ministries of Health of the four Central Asian countries.

Figure 1. Geographic Areas for Intervention against the HIV/AIDS Epidemic in Central Asia

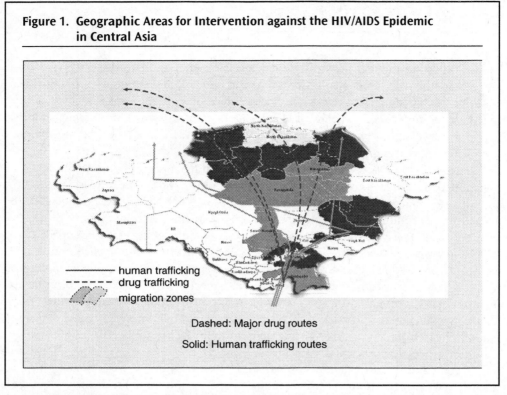

Source: Renton, Gzirishvili, Gotsadze, and Godinho (Forthcoming). *Epidemics and Drivers: Regional Challenge, Regional Response.* London: The Imperial College, DFID and the World Bank.

to all countries. NGOs are active in the region, and partner organizations and international NGOs have been providing significant technical and financial assistance. Despite growing regional commitment and resources to prevent and control the epidemic, there are, however, a number of issues that are not being adequately addressed.

Critical Gaps

First, groups such as truck drivers and migrants, who face higher exposure due to their mobility, are not presently covered; second, coverage of highly vulnerable groups such as injecting drug users (IDUs), commercial sex workers (CSWs), prisoners and youth at risk is still insignificant; third, treatment with anti-retroviral drugs (ARVs) is not yet available in most countries. Additional adequate policies for prevention and treatment need to be adopted; sentinel surveillance of HIV prevalence and surveillance of behavior are just beginning with assistance from CDC; and Government staff and NGOs need training in evidence-based clinical and public health practices and in program management.

These critical gaps, unless addressed promptly, will limit the effectiveness of the response to the evolving HIV/AIDS epidemic in Central Asia. While the potential scenarios of this epidemic are predictable, scientific evidence indicates that it can be slowed, stopped,

---

Critical Gaps

▦ **Coordination of different stakeholders** at national level is weak, and at regional level is almost non existent. Country Coordination Mechanisms have yet to clearly take the lead of the implementation of national strategies and programs, and coordinate the inputs of different stakeholders, including NGOs.

▦ **Inadequate surveillance and monitoring and evaluation systems** do not allow for effective planning and decision-making. Ongoing improvements in surveillance are establishing a viable base for crucial future second generation surveillance and outcome monitoring and evaluation, but require further support. There are few impact assessments of the efforts by national and international organizations to fight the epidemic.

▦ **Regional threats, or future drivers, of the epidemic** (drug-trafficking, trafficking of women, and migration) have not yet been adequately addressed.

▦ **Coverage of highly vulnerable groups** (IDUs, CSWs, MSM) by preventive services is below 15 percent, and is not expected to rise above 25 percent with existing resources. The prison population and migrant population are in general not covered by national and donor-funded programs. Only about half of the youth at risk will be covered with available resources, while it is recommended that at least 80 percent be covered for adequate epidemic control. There are only a few cases where pilot project initiatives have been expanded to national level.

▦ **Limited capacity to expand interventions.** The public sector lacks management and planning capacity to expand prevention activities and contract NGOs. Lack of resources for commodities and lack of skilled human resources and scalable project designs compound the problem. Implementation is led by international NGOs, which limits sustainability and reduces resources, and coordination between NGOs remains poor. In addition, there is little involvement of the private sector, municipalities and local communities on HIV/AIDS prevention in Central Asia.

▦ **The response to the four epidemics**—drug use, HIV/AIDS, STIs, and TB—is not integrated. Strengthening vertical structures will not contribute to a sustainable solution. Lack of integration and/or coordination among the National Drug Control Agencies, AIDS Centers, TB Institutes, Dermatological and Venereal Diseases Dispensaries and Narcology Departments; and institutional capacity in these services is limited. There is resistance to developing effective services to meet changing epidemic and health systems circumstances. Increasing access to, and modernizing STI Services and Narcology Services are in some cases being actively blocked by the relevant professional groups.

---

or even reversed. Countries which act early in the course of the epidemic—for example, before HIV prevalence reaches 5–10 percent among injecting drug users—are most successful in stemming the tide of the epidemic. A window of opportunity exists now for the countries of Central Asia to take effective interventions to a regional scale commensurate with the threat that they face.

If initial activities are not quickly expanded to ensure appropriate coverage of the most vulnerable groups and hotspots, the HIV/AIDS epidemiological situation in Central Asia may have an impact on population and economic growth, while costs of treatment with antiretroviral drugs would not be sustainable. The study on the potential economic impact of the epidemic (*see* Appendix B) has shown that a slowdown in GDP growth and losses in GDP level may be accompanied by losses in effective labor supply, which would be worsened by negative population growth in some countries. Even in an optimistic scenario, in all three countries studied (Kazakhstan, Kyrgyz Republic, and Uzbekistan) GDP in 2010 would be up to about 1.5 percent lower (from −1.4 percent in the Kyrgyz Republic to −1.75 percent in Kazakhstan). Without intervention, the cumulative loss would rise to roughly 2 percent by 2015 (−1.69 percent in the Kyrgyz Republic, −2.19 percent in Kazakhstan, and −2.7 percent in Uzbekistan). Perhaps more significant for long term development, the uninhibited spread of HIV would diminish the economy's long term growth rate, slowing it down by 2015 by roughly 3 percent in Kazakhstan and in the Kyrgyz Republic, and by about 5 percent in Uzbekistan. In a pessimistic scenario, however, the magnitude of these estimates could be three to four times higher. The study also indicates that, at current prices, the costs of HIV treatment would not be sustainable by the public budget if the epidemic is not prevented, and/or treatment costs are not cut dramatically.

The Bank will continue to assist regional Governments overcoming some of the identified critical gaps in four different ways:

- by pursuing advocacy and policy dialogue conducive to increase political will to take early action to prevent and control the four overlapping epidemics;
- by carrying out further sector work that will increase the understanding about the four related epidemics;
- by assisting the implementation of a proposed Regional AIDS Control Project that would contribute to decrease the potential negative impact of a major HIV/AIDS epidemic on regional development; and
- by providing technical and financial support at country level to implementation of the national programs aimed at controlling the four epidemics.

Recommendations for Key Actions

Reaching a political and social consensus on timely implementation of HIV/AIDS Strategies in Central Asia. Advocacy, communication, and participation activities have to be undertaken by Governments, NGOs, and international organizations to increase the awareness of policymakers, media, and the general public about the need to scale up initial actions; to facilitate the participation of various stakeholders—highly-vulnerable groups, vulnerable groups, and youth in general, decisionmakers, media, public sector, NGOs and private sector, and international NGOs and funding organizations—in the decisionmaking process, planning, implementation, and evaluation of key actions.

HIV/AIDS Program Coordination.   Clear leadership at the highest level of the National AIDS Programs would increase the chances of early prevention of HIV/AIDS in Central Asia. The implementation of National AIDS Programs, Global Fund grants, and the proposed Regional AIDS Project to be financed by IDA and DFID grants, and supported by UNAIDS, would benefit from the direct involvement of Presidents and Prime Ministers of Central Asia countries. The established Country Coordination Mechanisms, which include Government, NGOs and private sector representatives, should take the strategic lead of the implementation of HIV/AIDS National Programs. Under the leadership of the Country Coordination Mechanisms, intersectoral cooperation between regional Drug Control Agencies, Migration Offices, Narcology Services, and AIDS Centers should be promoted and supported.

Strategic and Policy Development. The legal framework should foster an enabling environment by reducing barriers that contribute to the high incidence of the disease. Program implementation would be facilitated by the adoption of a legal framework in each country that would: (i) protect the rights of people living with HIV/AIDS, including anti-discrimination laws; (ii) facilitate prevention work, such as decriminalization of practices associated with higher risk of HIV/AIDS; and (iii) increase access to necessary, confidential medical care, which includes policies on use of anti-retroviral drugs. The legislative and regulatory frameworks should be reviewed to enhance and modify police behavior towards highly vulnerable groups. The regulatory framework should also include policies on use of antiretroviral drugs following available international evidence and best practices to prevent the advent of drug resistance to ARV.

Surveillance and Monitoring and Evaluation. The ongoing regional program to improve sentinel and second-generation surveillance of HIV/AIDS with assistance from USAID/CDC should be further supported, technically and financially, by Governments and international donors. The UN-recommended principle of one M&E system per country should be followed, which requires coordination among different stakeholders financing and implementing programs. This coordination should be undertaken in the context of the CCM.

Capacity Building. Training is an area in which the proposed Regional AIDS Project may make a significant contribution to building regional capacity to tackle the HIV/AIDS epidemic. Local and international NGOs should play a predominant role in the HIV/AIDS program's implementation. Capacity building for NGOs is a critical activity that will promote long-term sustainability of the programs and improve implementation. Efforts should be made to build public-private partnerships, and to involve municipalities and mobilize communities to participate in promotion and prevention efforts.

Regional Drivers and Coverage of Highly Vulnerable Groups. The proposed Regional AIDS Control Project would specifically focus on regional drivers of the epidemics of drug use, sexually-transmitted diseases, HIV/AIDS, and TB. Resources will need to be focused on epidemiological hotspots where sentinel surveillance suggests that the observed regional differences in notification are not artificial. Partnerships between Governments, NGOs and international organizations have allowed initial coverage of groups most at risk. These partnerships should be pursued to ensure scaling-up of prevention programs, especially among highly vulnerable groups, to reach a proportion of these (50–60 percent) that enables adequate control of the epidemic. Injecting drug users and commercial sex workers, along with prisoners, are currently the groups most at risk and, therefore, the most risky channel for HIV transmission. Preventing the spread of HIV among these groups is advisable to prevent subsequent sexual transmission to vulnerable groups that do not inject drugs, and/or are not partners of drug users.

Funding of HIV/AIDS Programs. Coordination of different stakeholders under the leadership of the Country Coordination Mechanisms (CCMs), would improve the efficiency and effectiveness of use of available funds. There must be significant investment in policy development, management and coordination capacity especially focused towards management of GFATM and other grants; fund disbursement by Governments to NGOs; and overcoming structural political and vested interests barriers to implementation. The proposed Regional AIDS Control project would not only contribute additional resources to enable civil society and regional Governments to tackle the epidemic, but would also establish a mechanism for sustainable management of available grant funding.

Report Structure

This report includes an introduction on the global and regional context of this epidemic; information on the study design; and information about the Bank's activities in Europe and Central Asia. This is followed by a section on key emerging issues, which includes analysis of the extent of the epidemic in Central Asia; of potential economic consequences of the epidemic; and of early actions in the region to prevent the epidemic. Recommendations on key actions to promote a social and political consensus on HIV/AIDS, and ensure appropriate early action on HIV/AIDS ends the first part of the report. The background studies that were carried out under this Study, which include the detailed analysis of key issues, are included as Appendixes.

CHAPTER 1

Introduction

The Global HIV/AIDS Epidemic

The AIDS epidemic has entered its third decade worldwide. The global HIV/AIDS epidemic killed more than 3.1 million people in 2004, and an estimated 4.9 million acquired the human immunodeficiency virus (HIV)—bringing to 39.4 million the number of people living with the virus around the world.[4] There were around 42 million people globally living with HIV/AIDS at the end of 2002 (UNAIDS 2002). HIV/AIDS is now the leading cause of death in Sub-Saharan Africa, and the fourth main killer globally. Life expectancy has been cut by more than 10 years due to HIV/AIDS infection in several countries (UNAIDS 2001). The increasing speed of the spread of the epidemic increases the importance of the problem. Current projections suggest that an additional 45 million people will become infected with HIV in 126 low- and middle-income countries between 2002 and 2010, unless the world succeeds in mounting a drastically expanded, global prevention effort.

The ECA Regional Situation

In recent years, the Europe and Central Asia (ECA) region has seen the world's fastest growing HIV/AIDS epidemic due to a sharp increase in injecting drug use (IDU). A number of recent studies have pointed at the urgent need for action to manage the spread of HIV/AIDS

---

4. UNAIDS (2004) provides estimates based on the best available information and gives boundaries within which actual numbers lie. Thus, the number of people newly infected with HIV in 2004 is between 4.3 and 6.4 million; the number of AIDS death in 2004 is between 2.8 and 3.5 million; and the number of people living with HIV/AIDS in 2004 is between 35.9–44.3 million.

and limit its impact on the economic and social situation of countries in this region (World Bank 2003; Godinho and others 2004; Novotny, Haazen, and Adeyi 2003; Gotsadze, Chawla, and Chkatarashvili 2004; Kulis and Chawla 2004; Godinho and others, Forthcoming).

Economic and political instability throughout Eastern Europe and Central Asia have led to the increased spread of HIV/AIDS. In addition, there is a concern that HIV/AIDS prevalence in the region is underestimated due to the high number of unreported cases. The unreliability of official statistics is due to the inefficiency of the surveillance system (Miller and others 2004), as well as the nondisclosure due to fear of the stigma attached to HIV/AIDS. Officially, the number of HIV infections in ECA has grown from less than 30,000 cases in 1995 to an estimated 1.5 million by the end of 2003, a 5,000 percent increase. However, the real number is estimated to be much higher. The vast majority of these reported infections are among young people, mainly among injecting drug users—IDUs (UNAIDS 2003). The predominant role of drug-injections in HIV transmission is the major difference between the HIV epidemic in ECA and other regions worldwide.

Throughout the region, Governments and civil society, in cooperation with international agencies and NGOs, have started working on developing HIV/AIDS strategies to respond to the challenges posed by this disease. The Bank has been working with a number of client countries and partner organizations in the region on the preparation of new interventions to address the challenges imposed by the HIV/AIDS epidemic.

Central Asia AIDS: Study Design

To address the impending crisis in Central Asia, the World Bank has initiated the study of drug trafficking and use, HIV/AIDS, STIs, and TB in this region. These studies have been

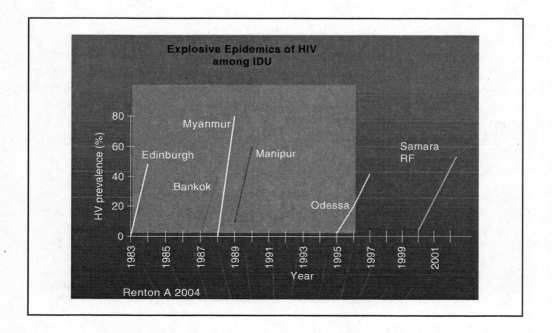

Box 1: Objectives of the Central Asia AIDS Study

The Central Asia AIDS Study aims at contributing to identify strategies for ensuring early and effective intervention to control the epidemic at national and regional level, considering priorities based on global evidence. The study also aims at informing the Bank's policy dialogue and the operational work to control HIV/AIDS in Central Asia; and contributing to building up the regional partnership between Governments, civil society, UN agencies, and multilateral and bilateral agencies to prevent HIV/AIDS and STIs in this subregion.

---

reviewing available data and evidence, gathering some original data, making projections for HIV/AIDS and mapping the four related epidemics in Central Asia.

The Central Asia AIDS Study has been carried out to contribute to the achievement of the global Millennium Development Goals (MDGs) (UN 2001), which have the following targets for HIV/AIDS:

- To reduce HIV infection among 15–24-year-olds by 25 percent in the most affected countries by 2005 and, globally, by 2010;
- By 2003, to have in place strategies that begin to address the factors that make individuals particularly vulnerable to HIV infection, including under-development, economic insecurity, poverty, lack of empowerment of women, lack of education, social exclusion, illiteracy, discrimination, lack of information and/or commodities for self-protection, and all types of sexual exploitation of women, girls and boys;
- By 2003, to develop multisectoral strategies to address the impact of the HIV/AIDS epidemic at the individual, family, community and national levels.

Specifically, the Central Asia Study aimed at answering the following questions:

(i) *What is the extent of the epidemic and likely impact of the HIV/AIDS epidemic in Central Asia?* These questions would be answered by the Central Asia HIV/AIDS and TB Country Profiles (Godinho and others 2004) and further update under this study on epidemiological data; and by modeling the potential economic impact of the epidemic in Central Asia.

(ii) *Have the regional Governments adopted reasonable and effective actions that could prevent the epidemic?* This question would be answered by in-depth policy analysis of existing strategies and policies, and of the existing legal framework, as well as by an analysis of the stakeholders involved in HIV/AIDS prevention and treatment, and institutional assessment of the capacity of the HIV/AIDS and STIs services and NGOs to prevent and treat the disease according to best practice.

(iii) *What is the regional and country-specific political economy vis-à-vis HIV/AIDS? What are the expressed and vested interests that may pose powerful obstacles to the implementation of existing strategies?* The stakeholder analysis and institutional assessment would allow the study audience to better understand some of the interests at play in the region, and how they can be overcome if they pose an obstacle to early and effective implementation of the HIV/AIDS Strategies.

(iv) *Would the Governments have the political willingness, and would the HIV/AIDS services and NGOs have the capacity to implement the strategies appropriately?* The stakeholder analysis and the institutional assessment would shed some light on these questions, and the communication strategy would contribute to raising the political and social will to take early action.

(v) *What is the funding available and expenditures on prevention and control of HIV/AIDS in Central Asia, and what are the existing gaps in financing and strategy implementation?* The stakeholder analysis and the institutional assessment would provide information on implementation of the approved strategies so far, and together with resource analysis, would indicate gaps in financing and strategy implementation so far.

(vi) *What should be done to contribute to reach a political and social consensus on timely implementation of the HIV/AIDS Strategies in Central Asia?* The proposed studies would serve as a basis to plan and implement advocacy, communication and stakeholder participation activities that contribute to reaching a social and political consensus on timely implementation of the HIV/AIDS Strategies in Central Asia, and specifically persuading Central Asia Governments to take early action to prevent the epidemic.

Additional studies were carried out with the following objectives:

(i) Update the epidemiological data about HIV/AIDS and STIs in Central Asia;
(ii) Estimate the potential epidemiological and economic impact of the HIV/AIDS epidemic in Central Asia;
(iii) Identify key stakeholders and their roles in controlling the epidemic;
(iv) Identify gaps in strategies, policies and legislation aimed at controlling the epidemic;
(v) Review funding available and expenditures on prevention and control HIV/AIDS in Central Asia;
(vi) Assess the institutional capacity, including of public health services and NGOs, to control the epidemic; and
(vii) Prepare the Bank's communication strategy on HIV/AIDS in Central Asia.

The study was carried out by reviewing existing statistics and literature on drug use, HIV/AIDS, STIs and tuberculosis in the countries under study; interviewing key stakeholders in the field; and discussing main issues and study findings with Government counterparts, NGOs and partner organizations in the field. Statistics and reports from the Government, NGOs and international agencies were reviewed. Several meetings with Government counterparts and representatives of international agencies took place, and NGO roundtables were organized in the countries under study.

This report includes the results of this second set of studies. The information on the epidemics included refers to four countries in the region: Kazakhstan; Kyrgyz Republic; Tajikistan and Uzbekistan. These countries are collectively referred to as the 'region' as no updated data are available for Turkmenistan. However, the stakeholder analysis and institutional capacity assessment include some information about Turkmenistan.

Central Asia HIV/AIDS and TB Studies and Operations

In 2001 and 2004, the Bank prepared Notes on HIV/AIDS in Central Asia, the first of which was updated and posted on the ECA website.[5] The first Note was prepared as a briefing document for the visit of the World Bank President to Central Asia, during which the Bank agreed with regional Governments that HIV/AIDS would be one of the three priority areas for the Bank's work in the region, along with water and energy. The second Note was prepared as a briefing document for the Bank's President advocacy work in the region.

Following the agreement reached during the President's visit in 2001, the Bank has: (i) pursued advocacy and policy dialogue conducive to increase regional political will to take early action to prevent and control the four overlapping epidemics; (ii) carried out sector work to increase the understanding about the epidemics and assist actions taken by regional Governments, NGOs and other stakeholders; (iii) assisted the preparation of a proposed Regional AIDS Control Project; and (iv) assisted the preparation of a public health component with HIV/AIDS, STIs, and TB activities under the Uzbek Health II Project.

On sector work, the Bank's Country and Sector Units agreed to carry out the Central Asia HIV/AIDS and TB Country Profiles, the Central Asia AIDS Study, and the Central Asia TB Study. Taken together, it is expected that these studies contribute to increasing the understanding of decision- and opinion-makers regarding the four epidemics and their potential human and economic costs, and facilitate early action to control HIV/AIDS. These studies were developed to inform regional decisionmakers, Bank management and

---

Box 2: Objectives of the HIV/AIDS and TB Studies in Central Asia

- Assess the extent of the epidemics, and the potential economic impact of an HIV/AIDS epidemic in Central Asia in the absence of appropriate early action;
- Assess whether early implementation of appropriate strategies to tackle the HIV/AIDS epidemic was taking place;
- Clarify the extent of the implementation of the WHO-recommended DOTS approach to control tuberculosis;
- Identify coverage gaps, and the underlying financial gaps and institutional capacity weaknesses that may constrain early implementation of appropriate strategies; and
- Make recommendations for action that would allow Governments and civil society, in cooperation with the Bank and partner organizations, to overcome some of the existing constraints.

---

5. www.worldbank.org/eca/ecshd or www.worldbank.org/eca/aids.

other stakeholders about the main characteristics of the epidemics in the region; to describe differences among the countries; to develop an understanding of the main issues related to the prevention of drug use, STIs, and HIV/AIDS, and the control of TB; and to make proposals for early action to prevent the four overlapping epidemics from further spreading throughout the region.

The Central Asia HIV/AIDS and TB Country Profiles (Godinho and others 2004) reviewed available epidemiological data; strategic and regulatory frameworks; surveillance; preventive, diagnostic and treatment activities; non-governmental and partner activities; and resources available in the five Central Asia countries. The study summarized main issues identified, and made recommendations for further study and action. The Country Profiles were based on review of statistics and reports existing up to December 2002, and on discussions with key stakeholders—Governments, NGOs, and donors—during several missions to Central Asia. The study summarized information available from Governments and partner organizations such as UN agencies, USAID, and OSI/ Soros Foundation.

The Central Asia AIDS Study was carried out as a follow up to the Country Profiles, to update epidemiological data (this study includes data from January 2003-December 2003, and when available up to December 2004); carry out economic projections of the epidemic; and carry out in depth reviews of stakeholders involved in early action to control HIV/AIDS in Central Asia, strategies recently adopted by Governments; resources that are being allocated to the implementation of these strategies; and institutional capacity to implement the strategies. A framework for a regional communication strategy on HIV/AIDS was also prepared.

The study team has carried out the mapping of regional corridors—the Northern Corridor and the Silk Route—for transport of people (CSWs, trafficked people, refugees, labor migrants, traders, truck drivers, travel staff, and so forth; Renton and others, Forthcoming) and goods (especially drugs); and mapping of drug use, HIV/AIDS, STIs, and TB cases.

The Bank has also carried out the Central Asia TB Study (Godinho and others, Forthcoming). This study aims at identifying constraints for implementation of appropriate programs to control TB in Central Asia, and suggest strategies to achieve target case detection and cure rates. The study includes a review of DOTS Programs implementation, and a

---

Box 3: Findings of the Central Asia TB Study

- DOTS implementation is progressing well but slowly, especially in Tajikistan;
- The situation in the penitentiary system in the countries visited is similar, with a very high case notification and TB death rate. However, prisons are not yet covered by DOTS or benefiting from funding available from GFATM and other sources;
- There is little monitoring of transfer of patients from the prison to civilian population;
- Tracer studies could help understand the movements of patients and the infection rates between prison-civilian transfers and civilian population;
- The additional burden of TB on the disability payment system should be studied as well. High rates of disabled patients are TB patients and the cost is high; and
- Authorities are unaware of the threat of the dual TB/HIV infection.

review of resources that have been allocated to TB control, including Government, donor and out-of-pocket contributions. The study makes recommendations for the Bank's policy dialogue and operational work in this area. It is also expected to contribute to building up of the regional partnership between Governments, civil society, UN agencies, and multilateral and bilateral agencies that have been working on TB control in the region.

An in-depth review of the Kazakhstan HIV/AIDS and TB Programs was undertaken in 2003–2004 (Cercone 2004). This review was conducted in the context of the policy dialogue between the Bank and the Government of Kazakhstan, and sector work that has been co-financed by both parties. The study includes (i) epidemiological review of TB and HIV/AIDS in Kazakhstan (ii) focus groups with PLWHA, TB patients and providers; (iii) TB and HIV/AIDS facility surveys; and (iv) a cost-effectiveness study of both programs. This review sheds additional light on issues of resource allocation, infrastructure, quality and patient and provider satisfaction.

Focus groups with people living with HIV/AIDS (PLWHA) have been carried out in Kazakhstan and in Tajikistan. In addition, the ECA External Department has carried out a Public Opinion Research in the Kyrgyz Republic (Box 4; Felzer 2004).

Box 4: Public Opinion Research in the Kyrgyz Republic

- Economy and jobs are overwhelming priorities for opinion leaders and general public. Health issues are attributed to economic woes.
- Health issues are considered very serious—they exist on the radar of opinion leaders and the general public (TB, HIV/AIDS, drugs).
- A focus on youth would resonate with all audiences.
- Complicated perceptions of HIV/AIDS: mix of denial and dissonance.
- Possibly, perceptions of HIV/AIDS confused with perceptions of TB, but both are of great concern. This is an opportunity to link the two.
- Excitement about direction of the country. General population believes Kyrgyz needs to be more open. This provides an excellent opportunity for discussion of HIV/AIDS.
- Outreach must reflect cultural norms.
- Dramatic behavior and attitude change toward the use of condoms is necessary.
- Opinion leaders welcome involvement of international groups.
- Opinion leaders recognize the need for a multi-sectoral approach to HIV/AIDS; it's not just about health.
- Youth highly trust information they receive about HIV/AIDS from parents, health/sexuality curriculum at school and their doctors.
- General public had the highest negative ratings for information coming from NGOs that is related to HIV/AIDS.
- Messages that resonate with general public and opinion leaders are: cost of prevention is less than cost of dealing with the disease, and protecting Kyrgyz's youth (they are vulnerable).
- Messages that do not resonate with general population are those which imply a sense of "doom" and over dramatization.
- Opinion leaders also recognize the need for more accurate accounting of the rising rate of infection, which they think could lead to support of a more aggressive approach.

Box 5: Proposed Bank-financed Operations on HIV/AIDS in Central Asia

In November 2003, the Bank initiated discussions with the Governments of Central Asia about the possibility of financing a **Regional AIDS Control Project** that would further assist implementation of the regional strategy to control HIV/AIDS. The proposed Regional AIDS Control Project would contribute to minimize the potential negative human and economic impact of a generalized HIV/AIDS epidemic, and complement country-specific programs and projects financed by Governments, the Bank and other partner organizations such as UNAIDS, GFATM, USAID and the OSI/Soros Foundation, among others. The project would be financed by IDA and DFID grants, and implemented with assistance from UNAIDS and USAID/CDC.

The **Uzbek Health II Project**, which is under implementation, includes a Public Health Component of $4.5 million. This component includes HIV/AIDS and TB subcomponents ($2.5 million) to be partly financed by an IDA grant. The TB subcomponent extends implementation of the WHO-recommended DOTS approach to two additional regions (oblasts). The AIDS subcomponent covers existing gaps in strategy implementation—the HIV/AIDS Strategy was prepared with assistance from UNAIDS, and was approved in 2003–, and complements funding by the Government, and Global Fund to Fight AIDS, Tuberculosis and Malaria (GFATM) and USAID grants for HIV/AIDS prevention and control.

On the operational front, the Bank has assisted the preparation of a proposed Central Asia Regional AIDS Control Project; and of the Uzbek Health II Project, which includes subcomponents on HIV/AIDS and TB.

The World Bank Role on HIV/AIDS in ECA

The World Bank has had a significant role in tackling HIV/AIDS globally in the context of the technical and financial support that it provides to Governments to implement appropriate multi-sector strategies. The Bank supports country-led efforts through non-lending services as well as credits and loans. In addition, the Bank is a co-sponsor of the global coalition against HIV/AIDS—the Joint United Nations Program on HIV/AIDS (UNAIDS) and a Trustee of the Global Fund to Fight AIDS, Tuberculosis and Malaria (GFATM). These organizations work in partnership with governments, NGOs, bilateral organizations and multilateral agencies to support country- and regional responses to HIV/AIDS. Specifically, the Bank has had a role on HIV/AIDS prevention and control in ECA in the following areas:

- *Regional Strategy.* The Bank has developed a regional strategy for its work on HIV/AIDS in 2003 (World Bank 2003).
- *Regional Sector Work.* There are variations among countries in terms of the size of the epidemic, income per capita, the political contexts, infrastructure and management capacities. Therefore, the Bank has been carrying out analytical work in the ECA region to assess the HIV/AIDS situation and its potential human and economic impact, including in Southeastern Europe (Novotny, Haazen, and Adeyi 2003; Godinho and others, Forthcoming), Central Asia (Godinho and others, Forthcoming), Georgia (Gotsadze and others 2004), and Poland and Baltic countries (Kulis and Chawla 2004).

Box 6: Bank-financed AIDS Control Projects in ECA

The Moldova AIDS Control Project supports the goal of the National Program for Prevention and Control of HIV/AIDS and STIs to reduce mortality, morbidity and transmission of HIV/AIDS, other sexually transmitted infections and tuberculosis. The Project is a component of the national TB/AIDS Program, which is financed in parallel from the following grants: an IDA grant of US$5.5 million for AIDS, a USAID grant of US$4.0 million for TB, and a US$5.2 million grant from the Global Fund to Fight AIDS, TB and Malaria (GFATM), both for AIDS and TB.

The Russia TB and AIDS Control Project ($150 million) supports the goal of the Government's Federal Program on Prevention and Control of Social Diseases to protect its population and economy from uncontrolled epidemics of TB, HIV/AIDS and other sexually transmitted infections.

The Ukraine TB and HIV/AIDS Control Project supports the Fourth Program on HIV/AIDS Prevention to reach the following objectives: to stabilize the epidemiological situation in the country; to reduce risky behavior among young people; and to reduce the social tension in the society and negative consequences of the epidemic. The total cost of the Project is $77 million, including a $60 million Bank loan, and $17 million from the Ukrainian Government.

- *Estimating the economic impact of HIV/AIDS at the country level.* Recent experience suggests that information on the likely economic impact of an unchecked epidemic could have a greater effect in securing the attention of policymakers regarding the need to take early action to control HIV/AIDS. This work has been carried out in Russia, Belarus and Moldova, and in Central Asia.
- *Refining estimates of human and financial resources needs.* Local capacity for developing and implementing programs varies enormously. Available information indicates a substantial gap in the necessary resources for effective interventions on a large scale. Therefore, the Bank co-financed with the UNAIDS Secretariat, the development of a Directory of Technical and Managerial Resources to enable countries to gain better access to high quality technical assistance; and a study of the incremental resource requirements for HIV/AIDS programs in ECA (UNAIDS and World Bank 2003).
- *Promoting a supportive policy environment.* With UNAIDS and other partners, the Bank is building support among key opinion leaders and elites for a dynamic HIV/AIDS control program. As this is particularly difficult due to the stigma attached (social, cultural, and political), the Bank carried out public opinion research studies in Albania and the Kyrgyz Republic (Felzer 2004).
- *Financing investments on HIV/AIDS control.* Given the relatively early stage of the epidemic, highest priority and Bank financing have been directed towards targeted interventions to prevent further transmission of the virus.

CHAPTER 2

Key Emerging Issues

Central Asia has been confronting four overlapping epidemics—drug use, sexually transmitted infections (STIs), HIV/AIDS, and TB—mostly having youth at its center. The drug use, HIV/AIDS and STIs epidemics mainly affect young people, while the TB epidemic affects people in their more economically productive years. Although the number of identified cases of HIV in Central Asia is still very low, the growth rate of the epidemic—from about 500 cases in 2000 to over 12,000 in 2004—is cause for serious concern. Central Asia lies along the drug routes from Afghanistan to Russia and Western Europe, and it is estimated to have 500,000 drug users, of which more than half inject drugs. There is a risk of major growth in the HIV/AIDS epidemic because of the risky practices reported by injecting drug users (IDUs), the high prevalence of sexually-transmitted infections (STIs), and increases in both commercial sex work (CSW) and labor migration to countries with higher prevalence of HIV/AIDS, such as Russia.

Current and future epidemics of HIV are and may continue to be driven by: a) explosive growth in injecting drug and commercial sex work use throughout the region; b) concurrent epidemics of STIs; c) economic and political migration; d) reduced capacity of governments/civil society to implement effective preventive responses; and e) low levels of awareness of HIV and STIs and of knowledge about risk behaviors and protection. These conditions in turn arise from economic decline since independence, as well as high volumes of drug transit through the region and growth of local consumer markets for these drugs.

Therefore, the countries of Central Asia are hyper-vulnerable to a serious crisis of HIV/AIDS over the next 20 years. Without concerted action, we may expect to see the rapid development over 4–5 years of an HIV epidemic concentrated among injecting drug users, and achieving very high prevalence levels in this group; followed by a generalized epidemic, developing over 15–30 years, with sexual transmission as the predominant mode.

This would follow the pattern of the epidemic in other regional countries such as Russia, Ukraine, and Moldova.

Much remains to be done, even though Governments and NGOs—with assistance from UNAIDS and other UN agencies, bilateral organizations (such as USAID, KfW, and DFID), and international NGOs (such as the Soros Foundation)—have been taking early appropriate action to control the epidemic. Additional adequate policies for prevention and treatment need to be adopted; active surveillance (sentinel surveillance and second-generation surveillance) is just beginning with assistance from the CDC; vulnerable groups such as truck drivers and migrants are not presently covered; coverage of highly-vulnerable groups such as injecting drug users (IDUs), commercial sex workers (CSWs) and prisoners is still insignificant; and treatment with anti-retroviral drugs (ARVs) is not yet available in most countries. On the institutional side, the mechanisms established to successfully obtain grants from the GFATM, are not functioning as leaders of the fight against the epidemic. No integration or collaboration exist between Drug Control Agencies, Ministries of Health, Interior, Justice and Education services dealing with the epidemics, and NGOs working with highly vulnerable and vulnerable groups.

The Extent of the Epidemics in Central Asia

Government estimates suggest that HIV prevalence among IDU remains below 2 percent and among pregnant women below 1 percent. However, one third of all identified cases were detected in 2003 alone, reflecting the very rapid increase in notification rates between 2000 and 2003—threefold in Kazakhstan; ninefold in the Kyrgyz Republic; 17-fold in Tajikistan and 16-fold in Uzbekistan; reaching in 2003 rates per 100,000 of 4.5 in Kazakhstan, 3.1 in the Kyrgyz Republic, 0.7 in Tajikistan, and 7.4 Uzbekistan. The male:female ratio was greater than 4:1 in all countries. In Tajikistan, the number of registered cases doubled in 2003, but in the first month of 2004 alone, the number of registered cases increased by more than 25 percent. The estimated prevalence rate among prisoners in Tajikistan and in the Kyrgyz Republic is around 8 percent. Within countries, there are marked geographical concentrations of HIV reported cases, with the Pavlodarskaya Oblast, Osh and Tashkent affected particularly hard.

Table 1. Newly-Diagnosed HIV Infections in Central Asia

	Up to 1996	1997	1998	1999	2000	2001	2002	2003	2004	Total
Kazakhstan	79	437	299	185	347	1,175	735	746	699	4,702
Kyrgyz Republic	19	2	6	10	16	149	160	132	161	655
Tajikistan	2	1	1	0	7	34	30	42	NA	117
Turkmenistan	—	—	—	—	—	2	—	—	NA	2
Uzbekistan	38	7	3	28	154	780	2,000	1,836	2,016	6,862
Central Asia	138	447	309	223	524	2,140	2,925	2,756	NA	12,338

Source: Ministries of Health of Kazakhstan, the Kyrgyz Republic, Uzbekistan, and Tajikistan (2004).

Surveillance data based upon compulsory notification are available but our ability to draw inferences from these is limited due to changes over time in testing policies. However, no reliable HIV sentinel surveillance data are available, and attempts to estimate prevalence among highly vulnerable groups (IDUs, CSWs, prisoners) have been confounded by technical difficulties. However, the CDC has been assisting the Government of Kazakhstan carrying out sentinel surveillance, and results are expected to be made public in the near future.

At the end of 2003 8,078 cases of HIV infection were reported in the region, 4,001 in Kazakhstan; 362 in the Kyrgyz Republic; 119 in Tajikistan and 3,596 in Uzbekistan. Of these, over 75 percent were notified as having been acquired through IDU. These figures certainly considerably underestimate the true number of cases in these countries; and reflect testing policy more than real prevalence. In particular, it should be noted that in Tajikistan HIV testing is only now becoming widely available; and in Uzbekistan there are over 5,000 HIV positive cases awaiting confirmation.

Although sexually transmitted infections incidence rates have stabilized in most countries, official rates are still quite high in Kazakhstan (over 100/100,000) and Kyrgyz Republic (around 50/100,000). Furthermore, the proportion of injecting drug users among HIV/AIDS cases has been decreasing, which suggests that sexual transmission is increasing. Therefore, the stabilization of STIs rates may reflect decreased access and/or notification rather than a real decline in the prevalence of these diseases.

Sexually-transmitted diseases other than HIV are important for two reasons. First, a person with a STI is both more likely to transmit HIV sexually (during any sexual coupling event) or more susceptible to acquire HIV, where the coupling is between HIV discordant partners. Second, high incidence rates of STI in a population are a marker for high underlying incidence of unprotected sexual activity, and sexual mixing patterns conducive to

STI/HIV Interactions	High STI Prevalence	Low STI Prevalence
No IDU harm reduction	1° explosive IDU epidemic 2° larger sexually transmitted epidemic	1° explosive IDU epidemic Smaller and slower 2° sexually transmitted epidemic
Successful IDU harm reduction	Contained IDU epidemic Smaller and slower 2° sexually transmitted epidemic	Contained IDU epidemic Very small and slow 2° sexually transmitted epidemic

Renton A 2004

HIV transmission. No sentinel surveillance data are available, but syphilis occurrence has been consistently estimated through passive surveillance. This shows that the region, like most of the CIS, has seen major epidemics of syphilis since the 1990s. The peak in 1998 registered over 20,000 cases of syphilis notified in the Kyrgyz Republic, Uzbekistan, and Tajikistan, with respective rates per 100,000 of 167, 47, and 24. Although rates had fallen by 2003, they remain 10–20 times higher than those observed in Western European countries, pointing to a very substantial underlying burden of STI incidence and prevalence in these populations. When geographical and age concentrations are taken into account, syphilis notification rates approach 1 percent among younger age groups.

Finally, notification of TB cases in Tajikistan and Uzbekistan jumped, respectively, by 50 and 40 percent in the last 5 years. Although there is not yet a significant overlap between HIV/AIDS and TB cases, this situation is expected to change in the future, as TB is the main opportunistic infection in AIDS cases. Despite the scaling up of the DOTS approach that has been occurring throughout these countries, the number of cases of TB may further rise in the future, as a consequence of the increase in AIDS cases. Therefore, preventing an HIV/AIDS epidemic also contributes to prevention of further increases in TB.

Risk Environment and Behavior

Drug trafficking and injecting drug use continue to increase throughout Central Asia—along the so called Northern Corridor that links Afghanistan to Russia through Central Asia. Consequently, HIV/AIDS incidence and prevalence will continue to grow. The economies of all countries in the region experienced a period of steep economic decline during the

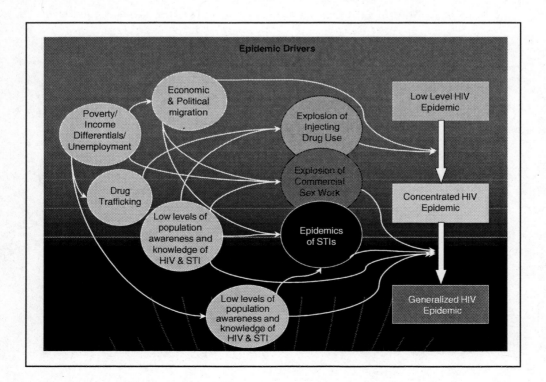

1990s, with destruction of jobs, public services and livelihoods. Over the same period, there was a rapid growth in the production of opium in Afghanistan, with UNODC (2001) estimating that in 2000, 75 percent of the world heroin supply was coming from poppies cultivated in Afghanistan, with around half of this exported through Central Asia.

Much of Afghanistan's opium production is refined into heroin and is either consumed by a growing regional population of drug users in Afghanistan, Pakistan, Iran, Turkey, and Central Asia (estimated 70–80 percent of total production); or exported, primarily to Western Europe (estimated 20–30 percent of Afghan production, and 85–90 percent of European consumption of heroin). Most of the drugs are transported by road from Afghanistan to Central Asia, CIS countries, and Western Europe, or alternatively, to Turkey, Balkan countries, and Western Europe. It takes around 10 kg of opium to produce one kg of heroin. In 2002, UNODC assessed the Afghan opium crop to be in the region of 3,400 tons.[6]

The significance for the region is huge, with between 30 and 50 percent of Tajikistan's economy estimated to be linked to narcotics trafficking. Seizures of drugs in Tajikistan have increased from 11 kilos in 1991 to 9 tons in 2003, of which almost 6 tons were of heroin, which shows the steep increase in drug production and distribution through Central Asia in 12 years. The number of registered drugs users in Tajikistan increased from less than 1,000 in 1996 to almost 7,000 in 2003, of which over 100 have been identified as infected with HIV/AIDS.

With transit and trafficking, local markets have developed; and with them an explosion of injecting drug use in all countries of the region. Although the true scale of opiate use, addiction and injection is difficult to estimate, current estimates of the number of injecting drug users in Kazakhstan, the Kyrgyz Republic, Uzbekistan, and Tajikistan vary between 300,000 and 410,000. That drug use has risen exponentially is confirmed by data from the State Narcology Services, with the Kyrgyz Republic and Kazakhstan seeing five-fold increases in the number of registered drug users between 1990 and 2003; Uzbekistan seeing an eight-fold increase since 1991; and Tajikistan a doubling over the two years 1999–2001. Male:female ratios vary between 18:1 and 10:1 in 2003; and around two thirds of registered users were IDU. Examination of the age-sex distribution of drug users reveals a strong clustering among younger men and in urban centers associated with drug trafficking transit points. Rates of registration for drug use among young men in Osh, in the Kyrgyz Republic, were estimated at 2 percent (2003), and in Dushanbe, Tajikistan, at 3.5 percent (2003). Given that the number of registered users will be only a fraction of actual users, the scale of this problem among young men and its potential future impact on the countries can be clearly appreciated.

Risk behaviors among injecting drug users have been found to be at high levels in these countries. Although inevitably data from surveys become rapidly out of date, all countries have reported high frequency of injection; low rates of sterile syringe use; high rates of sharing injecting equipment; and low rates of condom use with sexual partners.

Rapid assessments (UNAIDS 2002a, Uzbek CCM 2003, Tajik CCM 2002, Kyrgyz Republic CCM 2002, Kazakh CCM 2002) and estimates of the numbers of commercial sex workers (CSW) have been carried out in recent years. Estimates of the minimum number of CSW in each country are as follows: 50,000 in Kazakhstan; 5,000 in the Kyrgyz

---

6. The information in this section was provided by regional Drug Control Agencies and UNODC.

Republic; 5,000 in Tajikistan; and 20,000 in Uzbekistan. Rates of reported condom use are very low, and of previous history of sexually transmitted infection are high. One study in the Kyrgyz Republic found syphilis prevalence of over 30 percent in CSW attending a special STI clinic for the first time. Average numbers of partners per day are reported at around two, suggesting these women are having unprotected sex with hundreds of men each year. There is some evidence that the overlap between CSW and IDU is increasing.

There are high levels of migration in the region, which have been documented through the ongoing mapping study. This includes: ethnic migration, refugee flows, rural urban migration and external labor migration (including shuttle migration). These last two categories, in particular, are likely to be important in driving the HIV/AIDS epidemic in Central Asia. First, economic migration from the region is frequently into the Russian Federation. Russia itself is currently experiencing a major epidemic of HIV infection, largely concentrated among IDU (of whom females are commonly also CSW) but increasingly also sexually transmitted. Shuttle economic migrants are likely to be exposed to both sexual and IDU associated transmission while in Russia, thereby importing infection into their home country when they return, and potentially seeding this into local populations by sexual and drug injecting activity. Concentrations of existing cases of HIV are found in urban centers, thus exposing internal migrants to both injecting and sexual risks.

Social taboos concerning homosexuality have played a large part in marginalizing men who have sex with men (MSM) and in making reliable information about the numbers of MSM in the region or risk behaviors among this group hard to assess. Most men in this group are forced to hide their sexual behavior out of fear of persecution and prosecution, making it difficult for them to obtain information on issues such as safe sex and HIV/AIDS. One survey in Almaty city reported that condoms are used by MSM in only 20 percent of cases; and that that there are substantial rates of STI (25 percent) and drug use (10 percent). The Government of the Kyrgyz Republic recently estimated that there may be 30,000 MSM in the country, with 5,000 estimated to be living in Bishkek. There is undoubtedly a number of men who have sex with men in Uzbekistan, but this risk group is the most stigmatized and least understood. A 1997 situation assessment in Tashkent suggested that HIV/AIDS was not a major concern for this group, even though this group reported high levels of STI infection and low levels of condom use.

Prisons are an important part of the dynamic of HIV infection in the region. According to official statistics from the Uzbek Interior Ministry, about 12 percent of prisoners in 2000 were jailed for a drug-related crime, and the HIV epidemic in prisons is growing. The first case of HIV was registered in 1998. Nineteen cases were detected in prisons in 1999; 15 cases in 2000; 45 cases in 2001; and around 200 cases in 2002. Among 419 Kyrgyz citizens registered HIV positive by the end of 2003, 56 percent were identified among the prison population with an estimated HIV prevalence of 776 per 100,000, and of syphilis of 3,500 per 100,000. A recent rapid assessment (RAR) among male and female prison inmates in Tajikistan reports considerable risks for HIV transmission in Tajik prisons, as well as considerable numbers of imprisoned IDUs who may have acquired HIV infection outside prison. Some risk practices such as tattooing are common. Other risk practices such as injecting drug use are not as widespread, although 33 percent of those who had ever injected reported having done so in prison.

The Potential Economic Consequences of an HIV/AIDS Epidemic in Central Asia

This study carried out a modeling exercise to estimate the potential economic impact of the epidemic in Central Asia. The study includes a description of the model that has been developed following earlier work in the Russia Federation, but taking into account the specificity of the situation in Central Asia. Epidemiological and economic data from Kazakhstan, Kyrgyz Republic and Uzbekistan were used to estimate the potential economic impact of the epidemic in those countries. Epidemiological and economic data for Tajikistan and Turkmenistan are not available. The model can, however, be used when more reliable data become available for these countries.

This exercise was carried out to provide decisionmakers with scenarios (designated here as optimistic and pessimistic scenarios) of the potential impact of a generalized epidemic if no decisive action is taken. These should, therefore, be taken as scenarios and not as projections of the present situation, in which the epidemic is still concentrated in some well defined groups and early action is being undertaken by civil society and Governments.

The results are quite similar to those obtained by the Russian study. In the Russia Federation, it was estimated that, in an optimistic scenario, mortality rates would increase from 500 per month to 21,000 per month in the period 2005–2020, and the cumulative number of HIV infected individuals would raise from 1.2 million to 5.4 million during the same period. The Russia study estimated that, in what concerns the economic impact, uninhibited spread of HIV would diminish the economy's long term growth rate, taking off half a percentage point annually by 2010 and a full percentage point annually by 2020.

To better understand the mechanics and dynamics of HIV development, the Russia case was used as a reference point and forecasting device. Furthermore, the Russian experience sheds some light upon general patterns of HIV/AIDS infection in Central Asian countries. For a long time, Russia was known as a country of low prevalence of HIV-infection. The regular analysis of data showed that the first group of HIV infected Russians contracted HIV through sexual contacts with African and North Americans in the beginning of the 1980s (Pokrovsky 1996). The first case of a HIV positive Russian citizen was diagnosed in 1987. Presumably, in

---

Box 7: Potential Epidemiological and Economic Impact of HIV/AIDS in Central Asia

The study suggests that HIV in Central Asia may have a far-reaching impact on the economic development of the region if adequate and effective prevention activities are not ensured. A slow-down in GDP growth and losses in GDP level may be accompanied by losses in effective labor supply, which would be worsened by negative population growth in some countries. The study also indicates that, at current prices in the region, the costs of HIV treatment would not be sustainable by the public budget if the epidemic is not prevented, and/or treatment costs are not cut dramatically. As a policy implication, decisionmakers are advised to launch prevention programs, especially among highly vulnerable groups. Injecting drug users (IDU) are currently the group that is most at risk and, therefore, the most risky channel for HIV transmission. Preventing the spread of HIV among IDU is advisable to prevent subsequent sexual transmission to vulnerable groups that do not inject drugs.

the following two to three years, the HIV virus was actively transmitted through sexual contacts and detected in circles close to this original group of HIV-positive Russians.

Until mid-1990s, the virus slowly spread among heterosexuals and homosexuals alike, with approximately 100–200 new cases registered every year (while approximately 20 million persons were tested annually). By the end of 1995, the first cases were registered among intravenous drug users, and HIV began to spread rapidly, reaching 86,000 cases by the end of 2000, and 242,888 by June 2003. According to the Federal AIDS Center, Russia has the highest HIV growth rate in the world, except for Ukraine. In 2001, the number of registered cases was 88,422, twice as much as the total number of cases registered since 1987. Most recently (end of 2001 onward), heterosexual contacts took the lead again as the main source of infection, and the epidemic increasingly became a nationwide threat. A closer look at Russian data suggests that the time profile of the development of the HIV epidemic in Russia follows the exponential pattern, and this trend is likely to continue at least in the short-run. (See Appendix B for details.)

Similar research using Kazakh, Kyrgyz and Uzbek data reveals patterns of HIV growth strikingly congruent to what has been observed in Russia, despite poorer data quality. Nevertheless, all three Central Asian countries lag behind Russia, notably Uzbekistan and the Kyrgyz Republic: so far, they have not reached the stage when heterosexual HIV transmission prevails; also, HIV prevalence in the region is not as high as in Russia. However, taking Russia as a reference point, it may be concluded that in the absence of effective policy measures focused on controlling injecting drug use and prevention of HIV transmission from high risk groups (IDU, CSW, prisoners) to the rest of population, Central Asia countries are likely to replicate the Russian experience.

In all three Central Asian countries under study, the stage of slow HIV growth, at monthly rates of 0.01–0.02, was followed in the late 1990s (2001 in the Kyrgyz Republic) by a dramatic acceleration of HIV infection rates, with nearly a tenfold increase in the rates of growth, primarily among IDU. Nevertheless, in the near future, sexual transmission will likely take the lead and become the main source of infection, becoming increasingly difficult to identify highly vulnerable groups and control the epidemic.[7]

With no policy measures taken, and without preventive and antiretroviral treatment, two extreme scenarios (optimistic and pessimistic) of the epidemiological development in the region can be depicted. It is important to stress that these scenarios are not precise forecasts. Rather, they are benchmarks based on assumptions that are volatile over time. Among them are the long-term projections of the rate of growth of population, drug users, and GDP. Also, the multiplier that is used to estimate the number of actually infected individuals is estimated with uncertainty, notably in Kazakhstan and Uzbekistan. Regarding the fiscal costs of HIV treatment, the study used current costs of antiretroviral drugs, which are expected to continue decreasing in the near future.

---

7. In Kazakhstan, official statistics already suggest that there is an increase in the share of newly registered cases through sexual transmission (about 18 percent over the past eight month versus 10 percent on average over the whole observation period). However, these numbers should be treated with caution because, in September 2002, the Government abolished mandatory testing of prisoners, thereby lessening its surveillance basis. As a result, this may have an impact on statistics as the vast majority of HIV within the prison system are among IDU. Also, the increasing labor migration from low prevalence CA countries to Russia (that has much higher prevalence rates) will likely lead to an increase in the share of newly registered cases through sexual transmission.

More specifically, optimistic and pessimistic scenarios are based on different estimates of:

▪ *The rate of population growth* (low rate for the pessimistic case and high rate for the optimistic case). The growth rate brackets are different across countries and vary from [−0.5–0.1 percent] in Kazakhstan to [0.8 percent, 1.2 percent] in the Kyrgyz Republic, and to [1.8 percent, 2.4 percent] in Uzbekistan.

▪ *The rate of growth of drug users*, following the registered numbers officially reported (5 and 9 percent, respectively for the optimistic and the pessimistic scenario).[8]

▪ *The transmission rates of HIV across different groups* of the population. The transmission rate among drug users is 2 percent for the optimistic case and 5 percent for the pessimistic case—that is, one intravenous drug user is estimated to infect 2 to 5 other drug users per year. The transmission rate among non-drug users, in line with international estimates, has been set at 0.3 and 0.4, respectively; the rate with which HIV is transmitted from drug users to non-drug users has been kept at this same level;

Table 2. Economic Costs of HIV in Kazakhstan, Kyrgyz Republic and Uzbekistan (optimistic scenario)

	2010	2015	2020
Kazakhstan			
Monthly Mortalities (average)	11	45	120
Cumulative HIV (thousands)	0.20	0.40	0.80
% change GDP (compared to baseline)	−1.75	−2.19	−3.17
% change GDP growth (compared to baseline)	−2.59	−2.98	−3.43
% change Investment (compared to baseline)	−0.28	−0.36	−0.65
% change Effective Labor Supply (compared to baseline)	−2.02	−3.03	−3.06
Kyrgyz Republic			
Monthly Mortalities (average)	21	42	72
Cumulative HIV (thousands)	0.04	0.06	0.10
% change GDP (compared to baseline)	−1.40	−1.69	−2.34
% change GDP growth (compared to baseline)	−3.33	−3.44	−3.30
% change Investment (compared to baseline)	−2.00	−2.50	−2.86
% change Effective Labor Supply (compared to baseline)	−1.83	−3.45	**−4.07**
Uzbekistan			
Monthly Mortalities (average)	3	4	62
Cumulative HIV (thousands)	0.20	0.50	0.80
% change GDP (compared to baseline)	−1.59	−2.70	−2.91
% change GDP growth (compared to baseline)	−5.59	−4.75	−4.58
% change Investment (compared to baseline)	−0.08	−0.65	−0.71
%change Effective Labor Supply (compared to baseline)	−2.52	−2.99	−3.97

---

8. These numbers are based on estimates provided by the Federal AIDS Center in Russia and regional statistics. According to official statistics, in the first half of 2003 the number of drug users in Kazakhstan increased by 3.1 percent.

▓ *The multiplier* that is used to estimate the number of actually infected individuals from the number of registered HIV positive observations (this number is country specific and depends on the size and composition of tested sample). The scenarios have been calibrated for Kazakhstan with a multiplier of 2 for the optimistic case and 10 for the pessimistic case; for Uzbekistan with a multiplier of 2 for the optimistic case and 7 for the pessimistic case; and for the Kyrgyz Republic with a multiplier of 4 for the optimistic case and 6 for the pessimistic case.[9]

Without preventive measures and antiretroviral treatment, the human costs of HIV could be dramatic regardless the currently low prevalence rates. Due to the exponential nature of growth of HIV infection in an ignorant or indifferent environment, even in an optimistic scenario mortality rates in all three countries studied might increase dramatically. By 2020, the death toll might account for dozens of deaths a month; however, such long-term projections should be treated with caution as the model is based on assumptions that change over time. In the optimistic case, the cumulative number of HIV-infected individuals in Kazakhstan could rise to 20,000 in 2010, and 40,000 in 2015. The pessimistic scenario would result in substantially higher prevalence rates in Kazakhstan, with 170,000 infected in 2010 and 490,000 infected in 2015. For the Kyrgyz Republic and Uzbekistan, the optimistic/pessimistic estimates of the number of infected individuals would be, respectively, 4,000/10,000 and 20,000/100,000 in 2010, and 6,000/30,000 and 50,000/500,000 in 2015.

Furthermore, the hypothetical number of infected individuals who are in need of antiretroviral treatment could be used to estimate the potential pressure that the HIV epidemic might impose on the public health budget. The diversion of private and public resources, which otherwise would have been available to finance investment, into treatment and economically speaking toward consumption, comes at a cost to the economy, and this economic cost depends on the price at which antiretroviral treatment is available. At current prices, the costs of HIV treatment would not be sustainable by the public budget if the epidemic would not be prevented, and/or treatment costs were not cut dramatically. Based on the current regional costs for antiretroviral treatment of $9,000 per person per year, treatment costs in the pessimistic scenario—if paid in full—would provoke a severe

---

9. In Kazakhstan, with more than three-thirds of registered cases being among IDU, UNAIDS estimates that the real number of HIV positive cases is at least twice as high as the number of registered cases. According to official statistics, there are 47,241 registered IDU, while independent estimates place the real number closer to 250,000. However, the Government abolished mandatory testing of inmates in the country penitentiary system in 2002, thereby lessening its surveillance basis. In Uzbekistan, according to the information provided by the Uzbek AIDS Center, IDU are strongly prevalent among registered cases of HIV, with a share of 65 percent. According to an assessment conducted by UNODC in 2002, the total number of drug dependant people in Uzbekistan is estimated to be between 65,000–91,000, with only about 19,000 of them officially registered by the drug users service (Narcology Dispensaries). More than half of drug users injects drugs. The estimated total number of drug injectors (both occasional and drug dependant) in the country is about 200,000. Their injecting behavior in terms of sharing syringes and needles, and using human blood for the preparation of drug solutions, is extremely unsafe. Registered HIV cases are predominant in Tashkent City, Tashkent Province, and Surkhandariya Province with a prevalence of 1,100, 420 and 90 per 1 million population age 15–49, respectively. Thus, it is likely that the real number of HIV cases in Uzbekistan is much higher than the registered number. In addition, over 5,000 ELISA-positive blood samples have not yet been confirmed by Western Blot.

budget deficit in all three Central Asian countries. The Kyrgyz Republic would have to spend $4.4 billion in 2015 on HIV antiretroviral treatment alone, a figure that is comparable to the annual GDP of the country. Therefore, in the medium term, Central Asian countries will have to take preventive measures to slow down the spread of HIV epidemic, and negotiate prices for antiretroviral drugs to maintain a balanced budget.

Aside from the clearly visible negative impact of HIV on demographic variables (for example, a plain decline of the population due to increasing mortality) and budgetary expenditures (through excessive treatment costs), HIV will harm the quality of the labor supply, private and public investment, budget, and ultimately the GDP production and GDP growth. To estimate potential macroeconomic consequences of HIV, the study referred to a simple and robust neoclassical model of output production with labor and capital being factors of production. The study follows an interactive simulation approach designed to depict HIV/AIDS and economic developments, under various scenarios, which has been successfully probed to benchmark the economic consequences of HIV/AIDS in Russia (*see* Appendix B for technical discussion).

Under the assumptions discussed above, without preventive policies or treatment, effective labor supply (that is, labor supply proportionally adjusted for workers' productivity losses from being HIV-infected or/and addicted to drugs) would suffer a decline.[10] The magnitude of losses is comparable across countries and averages from 2 to 7 percent in 2010 and 3 to 11 percent in 2015, in the optimistic and pessimistic cases, respectively. However, the overall decline in Kazakhstan could be due more to a decline in the number of workers associated with negative population growth rate projections, while in the Kyrgyz Republic and in Uzbekistan, the effective labor supply would undoubtedly decline due to the productivity losses associated with the HIV infection rates among their work force. Since HIV adversely affects private investment (or savings) decisions and diminishes resources available for government investment expenditures, in all three countries *investment* would decline, although the magnitude of decline would vary across countries, and depends on the composition of public and private savings in the aggregate investment function.[11]

As a consequence of the decline in labor and capital inputs, GDP and GDP growth would be affected accordingly.[12] Even in the optimistic case, in all three countries GDP in 2010 would be up to about 1.5 percent lower (from –1.4 percent in the Kyrgyz Republic

---

10. It is important to distinguish the losses in effective labor supply from plain decline in the number of workers due to higher rates of mortality in certain age groups and areas, which can be partly compensated by substitution to capital.

11. Previous studies on the economic impact of HIV/AIDS revealed that household decisions to reduce savings or dis-save to meet increasing health care costs in a large measure contribute to a decline in capital accumulation. However, in many countries in ECA, an important share of health care expenditures are paid from the state budget. Also, the share of domestic savings varies across ECA countries, following the extent of development of local financial institutions. These data can be used to quantify the effect of HIV/AIDS on capital accumulation in a given country.

12. This study focus on GDP and GDP growth because these are immediate macroeconomic variables used by policymakers to depict the development of an economy. In the presence of a major epidemic, welfare indicators, such as GDP per capita, might appear to be less indicated. For instance, in the short run, the growth rate of GDP per capita may even increase following a severe decline in the population growth (see, for example, Greener and others, 2000, "The Macroeconomic Impact of HIV/AIDS in Botswana.").

Table 3. Impact of the Reduction in the Growth Rate of IDU
(Pessimistic scenario with growth rate of IDU changing from 9 to 2 percent)

	2010	2015	2020
	Kazakhstan		
GDP Levels			
with 9%	1.64	2.12	2.57
with 2%	1.66	2.17	2.64
Percentage gain	**1.22**	**2.36**	**2.72**
	Kyrgyz Republic		
GDP Levels			
with 9%	1.37	1.67	1.96
with 2%	1.39	1.7	2.01
Percentage gain	**1.46**	**1.80**	**2.55**
	Uzbekistan		
GDP Levels			
with 9%	1.19	1.35	1.52
with 2%	1.21	1.38	1.56
Percentage gain	**1.68**	**2.22**	**2.63**

to −1.75 percent in Kazakhstan). Without intervention, the cumulative loss would rise to roughly 2 percent by 2015 (−1.69 percent in the Kyrgyz Republic, −2.19 percent in Kazakhstan, and −2.7 percent in Uzbekistan). Perhaps more significant for long term development, the uninhibited spread of HIV would diminish the economy's long term growth rate, slowing it down by 2015 by roughly 3 percent in Kazakhstan and Kyrgyz Republic, and by about 5 percent in Uzbekistan (of the growth rate in the baseline "no-HIV case," which assumes that no disease will spread in the population). Note, however, that under the pessimistic scenario, the magnitude of these estimates will be three to four times higher.

As a policy implication, decisionmakers are advised to launch prevention programs, especially among highly vulnerable groups. Injecting drug users (IDU) are currently the group most at risk and, therefore, the most risky channel for HIV transmission. Preventing the spread of HIV among IDU is advisable to prevent subsequent sexual transmission to vulnerable groups that do not inject drugs. For instance, under the pessimistic scenario a change in behavior that would cut all transmission rates by a factor of four, for example, by limiting needle sharing or through sexual education programs, would improve economic performance in a moderate way by gaining from 1 to 2 percent of GDP level by the year 2015. The reason is that drug abuse and its negative effect on productivity (in Kazakhstan combined with population decline and its negative impact on labor supply) would continue unabated while the number of HIV positive individuals declines. However, such a change would dramatically reduce the HIV-related mortalities that will have far-reaching demographic consequences, especially in the context of population decline in Kazakhstan.

Furthermore, a softening of the decline in population growth in Kazakhstan can go a long way in compensating partially for the economic consequences of HIV.

Limiting the growth rate of drug users is among the most effective means of avoiding long term repercussions on economic growth and prosperity in the CA countries. The economic scope of this policy is comparable with—not to say exceeds—the positive effect of a reduction of HIV transmission rates, resulting in a gain of about 1.8–2.4 percent of GDP. This is explained by the fact that increased intravenous drug use not only accelerates the growth of HIV, but has additional negative effects on the aggregate productivity of labor, as the productivity of drug users is considerably below that of non-drug users. Again, under the optimistic scenario, the effect of the above policy measures will be less pronounced against a background of a milder negative impact of HIV spread.

Appropriate and Effective Early Actions to Prevent the Epidemic

Governments, NGOs and partner organizations working in the field have initiated appropriate early action to avoid a major HIV/AIDS epidemic. However the scale of these actions is too limited to appropriately cover the highly vulnerable groups (IDUs, CSWs, and prisoners), and vulnerable groups (young people at risk, truck drivers, migrants and others).

Four out of five regional Governments have approved and started implementation of appropriate HIV/AIDS strategies prepared with assistance from UNAIDS; and have applied for funding from the Global Fund Against AIDS, TB and Malaria (GFATM), which has been granted for HIV/AIDS to all countries. Partner organizations have been providing significant technical and financial assistance (Tables 8–10). However, weak capacity of the government(s) to coordinate donor assistance and orchestrate the efforts to combat the epidemic with the help of development partners, puts the current work at risk.

Table 4. Coverage of Highly-vulnerable and Vulnerable Groups

Country	Harm reduction			IEC			
	IDUs	CSWs	Inmates	High Risk Groups	General Youth	Labor Migrants	Military Servicemen
Kyrgyzstan	≈5%	≈2%	No	28%	60%	No	+
Tajikistan	≈6.4%	≈2%	No	54%	70%	No	++
Uzbekistan	6–17%	6–12%	No	37%	≈75%	No	+

Additional efforts are necessary to strengthen coordination mechanisms on a country and regional level. Weak national and regional coordination is just one contributing factor, which determines inadequate response. Coverage of highly-vulnerable groups is still well below desirable targets—for example, in the Kyrgyz Republic, USAID will cover 60 percent of youth with information, education and communication (IEC) activities, but less than 30 percent of highly vulnerable groups; and only 5 percent of IDUs will be reached by harm reduction activities, which are those that can most contribute to preventing the spread of the infection. Gaps in coverage are partly due to insufficiency of funding and partly due to lack of coordination among the different stakeholders.

Different stakeholders—highly-vulnerable and vulnerable groups that are the ultimate beneficiaries of policy and action in this area; civil society, decisionmakers, opinionmakers, and the international community—have interests that do not always coincide and, therefore, do not always contribute as intended to early prevention and control of the four overlapping epidemics. Lack of capacity (institutional and technical) among state institutions and local NGOs, which have to play a critical role in reaching out highly vulnerable groups, is another contributing factor that limits implementation of the agreed strategies. The number of local NGOs that work with high risk groups and provide critical services for prevention and control of HIV/AIDS, is still small, and these organizations require additional technical and financial assistance. Therefore, despite the availability of increasing (but still inadequate) resources to combat HIV/AIDS and STIs in the region, there are number of issues that are not being adequately addressed. These gaps threaten to undermine the effectiveness of the funds that are spent and could exacerbate the problems these countries face regarding HIV/AIDS and STIs.

HIV/AIDS Strategies and Programs in Central Asia

This study analyzed the HIV/AIDS Strategies and Programs that have been approved, and are under implementation in Central Asia, as well as regional initiatives by partner organizations: UNAIDS (2001a); GFATM (Kyrgyz Republic CCM 2002, Kazakh CCM 2002, Uzbek CCM 2003, Tajik CCM 2002); USAID (2002); and DFID (2004). The detailed analysis of the strategic and legal framework shows that the policy environment of all five Central Asia Republics regarding HIV/AIDS prevention still reflects the previous history of Soviet approaches to communicable diseases. The situation has changed considerably since the beginning of the HIV epidemic, but further policy support for tolerance, human rights protections, and appropriate medical and social support for HIV-related medical conditions is needed.

The Government of Kazakhstan has recognized the need to intervene to avert the epidemics, has put into place coherent strategies, and secured funds through international donors and the GFATM. However, significant barriers remain to delivering a timely response. Strategic plans in Kazakhstan call for an intersectoral approach and this appears to be quite well achieved at high governmental level. In 2002, sectoral strategic AIDS response programs for the period up to 2005 were developed by the Ministries of Health, Education, Defense, Interior, Justice, Culture, and Information. AIDS Coordination Committees were established at the ministries to implement strategic AIDS prevention and control programs. The Republican AIDS Center with technical and financial support from UNAIDS and other UN agencies, played a major role in this process, but the input of NGOs to this, and indeed the role of NGOs more broadly in the field is weak. The CCM, which was formed for the Global Fund grant application and implementation, successfully applied for grants for HIV/AIDS and TB, and meets on a regular basis. However, some institutions are concerned that the MoH does not have a strong interest in the HIV/AIDS program, and does not provide adequate funding. There are serious concerns among UN agencies and within some of the state bodies that resistance among narcologists and dermato-venereal diseases specialists to some of the innovations planned within the Strategic program will make delivery extremely difficult.

The Government of the Kyrgyz Republic has been active in grasping the significance of the epidemics of HIV and sexually transmitted diseases for the country. Although the central Government commitment to fight HIV/AIDS is in place, further advocacy is necessary to engage the Presidential Administration and national Government in the control of the epidemic. The Strategic Plan to control HIV/AIDS epidemic in the country was developed through a broad Government and NGO consultation process. Most NGOs specializing on work with IDUs, CSW, MSM, and other highly-vulnerable groups contributed to the development of this strategy along with public institutions. Despite strong ownership, significant barriers remain to delivering a timely response. These include: (i) inadequate resources to deliver interventions at scale; (ii) inadequate staffing levels and training in public health analysis and decisionmaking at all levels; and (iii) inadequate salaries at all levels to allow public health officials to adequately perform their public health functions rather than focusing on income generation.

The Tajik policy environment currently appears to be changing through a mix of the Strategic Program and GFATM Plan actions. The National Program on Prevention and Control of HIV/AIDS until 2007 establishes the National Coordinating Committee, and defines financing, multisectoral commitments, and program directions. Tajikistan's National Coordination Committee on HIV/AIDS and STI Prevention is led by the Deputy Prime Minister, and the importance of protecting IDUs from HIV infection is accepted at the highest levels, including the Ministry of Justice and Internal Affairs of Tajikistan. However laws criminalizing people who knowingly spread HIV or sexually-transmitted infections, as well as individuals who avoid medical examination or otherwise attempt to conceal their infection, still remain. These laws combined with police harassment and possible arrest for possession of even a used syringe, drive drug users underground. Actual responses have been rather uncoordinated and influenced by donor agendas, and therefore coverage remains low.

The Government of Uzbekistan has been steadily building its commitment and capacity to respond to HIV/AIDS. Most recently, the Government developed and approved the Strategic Program on Counteracting the HIV/AIDS Epidemic in the Republic of Uzbekistan for 2003–2006. However, there are also a number of negative factors within the risk environment. State structures concerned with prevention and treatment of infectious disease still play a role very much akin to policing infected individuals. Notably within the Dermatological and Venereal Diseases Service, militia are still involved in capturing segments of the population (particularly CSW) and bringing these compulsorily into the Dermatological and Venereal Diseases Dispensaries. There is an attitude of closure and secrecy in relation to the availability of official statistics describing HIV/STI and risk behaviors. The NGO sector exists, but is not flourishing or as energetic as in the Kyrgyz Republic. The Government has responded to the need for harm reduction projects by issuing a decree to set up a large number of 'Trust Points', which should deliver voluntary testing and counseling (VCT) as well as advice and harm reduction commodities. However, it does not provide significant support to NGOs in this work. These factors will need to be addressed if an effective scaled-up response is to be achieved. In addition low levels of knowledge about HIV/AIDS are likely to be an impediment to prevention.

Drug-related laws seem to shy away from specific criminalization for drug use, while making the possession of small amounts of illegal drugs a crime. This sets the stage for both repression and corruption. It also creates a situation in which injecting drug users (IDUs) are segregated from medical and social support systems, allowing HIV infection to become more and more concentrated until it bridges into sexual networks outside the IDU community. In terms of policy on IDU approaches, the widespread adoption of harm reduction approaches should be considered a top priority (Des Jarlais and Friedman 1994). These include non-specialized, decentralized, and more freely available substitution therapy for drug use. For this to occur, legislative change is necessary to liberalize the use of methadone and other substitution drugs. Narcology Centers should not be the only places authorized to provide this treatment. Needle exchange needs legalization and accompanying authority for providers to implement without fear for security. This approach is insufficiently described in all of the Strategic Plans reviewed.

Policy approaches to commercial sex work (CSW) suggest a need for decriminalization, both in terms of the definition of laws dealing with prostitution and enforcement practices. Gender issues are not addressed by the Strategic Plans, and this should be an area of concentration for policy work. Users of commercial sexual services are not prosecuted in general, while CSWs (most at risk for STI and HIV) are marginalized and isolated by police practices.

Policies to support expanded outreach medical treatment for STIs, IDUs, and young people may need further attention throughout the region. The specialized, medical approach to HIV/AIDS cannot be the only approach to reaching vulnerable groups; whether through legislation, funding, or expanded NGO support, decentralized and culturally appropriate facilities will require supportive policies in order to prevent HIV spread across bridging populations.

Box 8: Injecting Drug Use Interventions Related to HIV/AIDS

Demand side
1. Decriminalizing use (reducing prison population size)
2. Expanding treatment opportunities: GP or non-specialist use of methadone
3. Needle exchange
4. Condom social marketing
5. VCT expansion through peer counseling and outreach

Supply side
1. Strengthening penalties for trafficking
2. Financial incentives to offset trafficking in narcotics
3. Improved border protection and law enforcement

Table 5. Data on Antiretroviral (ARV) Therapy Policies and Funding

Country	Draft ARV Policy	ARV Policy Operational (date)	Bank Funds Support ARV	Other Funds Support ARV	Target Numbers for ARV Treatment by 2005
Kazakhstan	Yes (Children & expectant Mothers, currently; GFATM will expand)	Unknown	No	GFATM grant (03)	500
Kyrgyz Republic	No (GFATM provision for full coverage by 2007)	No	No	GFATM grant (03)	100% of those who need it ($n = 300$)
Tajikistan	No (GFATM provision for full coverage)	NO		GFATM grant (03)	
Turkmenistan	No (AIDS Strategy)	No	No	No	
Uzbekistan	Yes	No	IDA grant & credit but not for ARV (04) ($2 million)	GFATM grant (04)	100

Stigma against vulnerable groups and people living with HIV/AIDS (PLWHA) seems to be extensive in Central Asia. Thus, policies protecting human rights, confidentiality, and anonymous voluntary counseling and testing (VCT) need to be specifically addressed.

Two of the four countries of Central Asia that have obtained GFATM grants—Kazakhstan and Uzbekistan—have new anti-retroviral drugs treatment (ARV) targets for 2005 and 2007, respectively. Most of the health systems in ECA more or less guarantee treatment for infectious diseases. However, the costs of ARV so far have limited the reality of this guarantee to certain target groups. For example, in Kazakhstan, only children and pregnant women were covered by ARV treatment before the award of the GFATM grant. The key policy gaps related to ARV have to do with specific financing strategies: negotiations for equity pricing, protocols for treatment based on scientific evidence and international standards, monitoring of drug resistance, and improvement in laboratory support for ARVs are insufficiently addressed in the Strategic Plans. Data on antiretroviral (ARV) therapy policies and funding are presented in Table 5.

It appears as though a substantial investment in policy and legislative modernization is needed in each country. All Strategic Plans suggest the need for cross-sectoral collaboration and action. However, in reality, the territoriality of programs and jurisdictions is very difficult to overcome. The credibility and functionality of the National Coordinating bodies in each country will determine the success of the multi-sectoral activities.

Central Asia has been benefiting from substantial technical and/or financial assistance from UN agencies, bilateral agencies and international NGOs, and recently from Global Fund grants. UNAIDS recognizes the need for harm reductions strategies and legislative reforms. UNODC recognizes the need for improved drug treatment balanced with interdiction approaches, but there really seems to be a lack of commitment to reducing demand for drug use through liberalizing the criminal code. UNICEF stresses the importance of youth vulnerability, as well as the need to attend to children of AIDS victims (an issue marginally addressed in the Strategic Plans). USAID calls for improvements in surveillance, blood safety, and youth-oriented education.

Table 6. Groups at Risk, Their Needs and Current/Expected Coverage Rates[13]

Group	Size	Characteristics	Needs & Coverage
IDUs	466,000–494,000	High prevalence of HIV	Harm reduction (HR)
		Fast increasing in numbers	IEC
		Low awareness about HIV	Methadone Replacement Therapy
		Adverse behavior—needle sharing	VCT
			Expected coverage with the services is estimated at <5%
			IEC
CSWs	28,000–58,000*	Increasing numbers	Methadone Replacement Therapy
		Growing share of IDUs	Friendly clinics for medical services
		Low awareness about HIV	VCT
		Adverse behavior—unsafe sex	Condom distribution
		High prevalence of STIs	Expected coverage with the services is estimated at <5%
Prisoners	139,800–143,300	High prevalence of HIV	Harm reduction (HR)
		Low awareness about HIV	IEC
		Adverse behavior—needle sharing	Methadone Replacement Therapy
			VCT
		High chance of contracting TB along with HIV	Condom distribution
			Almost no coverage***
Migrants	870,000–920,000*	Frequently involved in risk behavior	IEC
			Harm reduction (HR)
		Low awareness about HIV	Friendly clinics for medical services
			Almost no coverage
At-risk youth[14]	730,000**	Low awareness about HIV	IEC through peer education sessions
		Risk to be involved in adverse behavior	Harm reduction (HR)
			VCT
			Coverage under DDRP will reach only 39 percent in 2007

*Does not includes Uzbekistan as data were not available; **Estimates of DDR program; ***Limited condom distribution; and pilot needle-exchange and MRT in prisons only available in the Kyrgyz Republic.

---

13. The coverage rates presented in the table are based on the assessment of available and projected donor funding.

14. The estimates for at-risk youth are based on information from PSI—DDRP.

Ultimately, the countries will have to decide for themselves how best to change national policies, but the evidence-base provides for substantial support for harm reduction policies and much more extensive substitution therapy. The evidence is still unclear as to the applicability of decriminalization of drugs as an effective HIV prevention strategy, but it is clear that current legislative approaches do not support effective interventions on IDU-related HIV prevention.

Political Economy vis-à-vis HIV/AIDS

Assessments of stakeholders and institutional capacity were undertaken to better understand an environment of rapid epidemiological and institutional changes; and to advocate for HIV/AIDS and to promote stakeholder participation. The main findings of these assessments are summarized below. Tables 6–10 include additional information.

The HIV/AIDS epidemic is rapidly growing in Central Asian countries. High levels of poverty, and the significant economic and social problems of the general population, coupled with low public spending in social areas, create an atmosphere in which society marginalizes at risk groups. The needs of these groups are hardly met, which significantly increases the risks of a more generalized epidemic. This may significantly affect the future economic and development prospects of these countries.

The groups most at risk are: (i) intravenous drug users (IDU), (ii) commercial sex workers (CSW), (iii) at-risk youth,[15] (iv) prisoners, and (v) mobile/migrant populations. The size of the groups at risk is up to two million individuals. Well-documented adverse behavior of high-risk groups creates an environment conducive to the spread of HIV.

Across the region coverage rates for individual risk groups remain very low. Current or expected coverage rates of highly vulnerable groups with preventive services are significantly below the proposed levels for effective epidemic control. Even in the best cases, the coverage rates are typically below 15 percent and are not expected to rise above 25 percent given existing Government, GFATM, and other resources. Moreover, there are only a few cases where pilot project initiatives have been expanded, or scaled-up to the national level.

Barriers to expansion and scaling up include competing policy priorities, and lack of funding and institutional capacity. However, the stigma attached to highly vulnerable groups such as IDUs and CSWs plays a significant role in the level of priority that decisionmakers and other stakeholders give to the four overlapping epidemics. Barriers include not only lack of resources for commodities; but also and very importantly lack of skilled human resources and generalisable project designs. The implementation of most activities has been almost entirely led by international NGOs thereby limiting the sustainability of the activities and reducing the amount of resources that are directly allocated to program interventions (rather than overhead and international TA). Moreover, coordination between agencies remains poor.

The prison system is lagging behind in the prevention of HIV/AIDS. Its weakness is attributable to several factors. In most countries, the system maintains the old soviet-type

---

15. For the purposes of this report, "at-risk youth" are those most at-risk of initiating injecting drug use, including: friends and family of injecting drug users; out-of-school and/or unemployed youth in drug communities; and other young people living in drug communities.

Table 7. HIV/AIDS Stakeholders in Central Asia

Stakeholders	Drug Epidemic	HIV/AIDS Epidemic	STI Problems	TB Epidemic
Beneficiaries				
▓ Highly vulnerable groups	Drug users	IDUs	Drug users	Poor
	CSWs	CSWs	CSWs	Prisoners
	Prisoners	Prisoners	Prisoners	
	At-risk youth	At-risk youth	At-risk youth	
	Migrants	Migrants	Migrants	
▓ Vulnerable groups	Youth	Youth	Youth	
	Drug users	PLWHA	STIs patients	TB patients
	Families	Families	Families	Families
▓ Patients				
▓ General public				
Providers				
▓ NGOs	Narcology Centers	AIDS Centers	DVDs	TB Institutes
▓ Public services	DCAs	NGOs	NGOs	Prison Healthcare
▓ Private services	Prison Healthcare	Prison healthcare	Prison Healthcare	
Decisionmakers				
▓ President	President	President		
	Prime Ministers	PM, DPM		
▓ Cabinet of Ministers	Deputy PMs	MoH, MoI, MoE, MoLSP, MoFA	MoH, MoI, MoJ	MoH, MoI, MoJ
	MoH, MoI, MoJ, MoE			
▓ Sector Ministries				
Opinion-makers	Low involvement	Low involvement	Not *adequately* addressed	Not *adequately* addressed
▓ Media				
▓ Advocacy groups				
Funding agencies				
▓ UN	UNODC	UNAIDS	UNAIDS	WHO/GDF
▓ GFATM	USAID	UN Agencies	WHO	GFATM
▓ IFCs	Soros	GFATM	UNFPA	USAID
▓ Bilateral donors		USAID, DFID	GFATM	KFW
▓ Int. NGOs		SDC, JICA		MSF
		Soros, AFEW		

Table 8. Early Action on HIV/AIDS in Central Asia Countries

	Kazakhstan	Kyrgyz Republic	Tajikistan	Turkmenistan	Uzbekistan
Year of Strategic Plan	NSP completed for 2001–2005	NSP completed for 2001–2005	NSP completed for 2001–2004	NSP being developed	NSP in process
Multi-sectoral body for coordination of response	Central and regional cross-sectoral committees chaired by Dep PM & Dep Governors	Republican Co-ordination Committee under the first Vice Prime Minister	National AIDS Committee established at the national and regional level. UN-TG effective.	Inter-Ministerial Task Force led by MoH fully operational. UN-TG actively assisting	Inter-Ministerial Task Force on priority communicable diseases established
Demonstrated high level of commitment	Highest level of commitment: President, Dep Prime Minister—chairs. Budget allocation not yet following strategy.	VP Chairs Committee Commitment but lack of unified state policy. Major gaps in resources & capacity Roles of GOV and NGO players clear	VP chairs Committee. Government faces serious financial constraints. Concern that it will be paper exercise.	Advocacy is needed	Creation of NACC in PM's office is initiated. Limited vision or coordination. Dedicated NGOs but dependent on key individuals
Working Technical Group	UNDP/UNAIDS, WHO, UNODC, WB, UNESCO, Soros, IPPF, Red Cross and Red Crescent, AIDS Center, STI Center	WHO, UNODC, UNDP/UNAIDS, WB, UNESCO, UNICEF, UNFPA, WHO, IOM Soros, IPPF, Red Cross Red Crescent, AIDS Center, STI Center, ADB	WHO, UNODC, UNDP/UNAIDS, WB, UNICEF, UNFPA	WHO, UNODC, UNDP/UNAIDS, WB, UNICEF, UNFPA, USAID, Peace Corps, MoH, National AIDS Prevention Center, National Youth Union	WHO, UNDCP, UNDP/UNAIDS, WB, UNICEF, UNFPA, USAID, MoH, UNESCO,
GFATM Application	$23,282,000 for 5 years	$17,073,000 for 5 years	$8,752,489 for 4 years	Government: ??;	$24,498,000 over 5 years
Other Financial Inputs	USAID $6.7 m prevention; CDC surveillance; PSI social marketing; UNICEF $4.5 m HIV/AIDS GOV $6.35 m (2002) undisbursed	GOKY $180,000 in 2001; UNDP & UNAIDS $250,000 UN, SOROS/OSI & loc govt fund harm reduction; DFID, Netherlands, Osh—$24,000 for condoms	Government: $ for infrastructure and labs; UNICEF: $6 m 2000–2004; UNDP, UNICEF, SOROS $ for vulnerable groups	USAID: $100,000: 2003 ADB??; UNICEF: $4.3 m 2000–2004	UN, USAID & OSI $1.5 m — 2001–2003; KfW DM5 m — Family Planning, condoms and contraception

Table 9. Key Elements of Country Strategies

Kazakhstan
- To stabilize HIV infection and prevent the spread of HIV from concentrated pockets to a generalized epidemic
- To decrease the number of young people being infected with HIV—reduce the vulnerability of youth
- To provide at least 80 percent of HIV infected people with medical and social programs in order to reduce contagion

Kyrgyz Republic
- To improve National policy related HIV/AIDS/STI problems in the Kyrgyz Republic
- To assure safety of provided medical services
- To reduce vulnerability of youth
- To reduce vulnerability of injecting drug users (IDUs)
- To reduce vulnerability of commercial sex-workers (CSW)s
- To develop IEC campaigns for prevention of HIV/AIDS
- To develop medical service provision for STI patients
- To prevent prenatal HIV infections.
- To provide medical and social support for HIV and AIDS infected patients and their family members.

Tajikistan
- To reduce the vulnerability of young people
- To reduce the vulnerability for IDUs
- To reduce vulnerability among CSWs and their clients

Turkmenistan
- To define HIV/AIDS/STIs policies, including revision of current legislation
- To develop early prevention of HIV/AIDS
- To prevent HIV/AIDS blood transmission
- To prevent sexual transmission of HIV/AIDS through safer sex behavior, provision of condoms and availability of STIs information, counseling and care
- To prevent mother-to-child transmission through provision of information and condoms
- To support people living with HIV/AIDS

Uzbekistan
- To integrate HIV/AIDS and STI issues into the key concepts of the Republic of Uzbekistan's development, through multi-sectoral collaboration
- To produce legislative reforms providing better access to prevention programs for high risk groups
- To implement prevention programs among groups with behavior associated with high risk of HIV infection
- To implement programs to increase awareness of population, particularly youth, about HIV/AIDS
- To create better accessibility, acceptability and quality of medical services related to HIV/AIDS
- To establish a national coordination mechanism to respond to the spreading of the HIV/AIDS epidemic

Table 10. Funding Available and Planned for HIV/AIDS Prevention and Control in Central Asia (thousands of US$)

Country	Total US$	2002	2003	2004	2005	2006	2007	2008	2009	2010
Kazakhstan										
Government	4,748,971	249,054	310,964	336,000	578,514	604,551	628,732	653,881	680,036	707,238
Partner Organizations*	14,304,975	165,611	1,622,754	3,316,110	5,240,500	1,350,000	1,350,000	1,140,000	120,000	0
Total funding for HIV/AIDS	*19,053,946*	*414,666*	*1,933,718*	*3,652,110*	*5,819,014*	*1,954,551*	*1,978,732*	*1,793,881*	*800,036*	*707,238*
*of which GFATM					2,518,010	3,983,000				
*Partner funding from 2006: USAID (until 2008)										
Kyrgyzstan										
Government	1,472,000	n/a	125,000	136,000	264,333	264,333	264,333	139,333	139,333	139,333
Partner Organizations*	22,528,688	323,735	677,525	4,827,690	5,823,311	3,146,714	2,617,429	2,617,429	1,247,429	1,247,429
Total funding for HIV/AIDS	*24,000,688*	*323,735*	*802,525*	*4,963,690*	*6,087,644*	*3,411,047*	*2,881,762*	*2,756,762*	*1,386,762*	*1,386,762*
*Partner funding from 2006: DfID (until 2008), USAID (until 2008), KfW, UNDP (until 2010)										
Tajikistan										
Government	855,584	455,584	400,000							
Partner Organizations*	15,638,365	201,735	1,436,385	2,678,272	2,952,897	2,940,857	2,728,218	1,970,000	730,000	0
Total funding for HIV/AIDS	*16,493,949*	*657,319*	*1,836,385*	*2,678,272*	*2,952,897*	*2,940,857*	*2,728,218*	*1,970,000*	*730,000*	*0*
*Partner funding from 2006: SDC (2006), USAID (until 2007), DfID (until 2008)										
Uzbekistan										
Government	1,826,333	455,584	770,749	600,000						
Partner Organizations*, **	22,455,518	278,590	2,439,916	2,682,750	5,290,832	5,114,715	4,548,715	1,798,000	302,000	—
Total funding for HIV/AIDS	*24,281,851*	*734,174*	*3,210,665*	*3,282,750*	*5,290,832*	*5,114,715*	*4,548,715*	*1,798,000*	*302,000*	*—*
*of which World Bank:	1,856,000			56,000	108,000	475,000	637,000	278,000	302,000	302,000
**other partner funding from 2006: USAID (until 2008), DfID (until 2008)										

Sources: Ministries of Finance and Health; international organizations including GFATM, 2004.

command and control military structure. However, in Kazakhstan, Kyrgyz Republic, and Tajikistan, prisons were transferred from the Ministry of Interior to the Ministry of Justice, while in Uzbekistan they remain under the MoI. The penitentiary system is constrained by punitive laws towards IDUs, CSWs, and MSMs, which do not freely allow needle-exchange programs, condom distribution and other harm-reduction and preventive interventions to take place in the prisons. Medical staff employed in detention facilities need training and support to change attitudes towards inmates.

The needs of the migrating population are only partially addressed throughout the region. The International Office for Migration (IOM) is the agency working on HIV/AIDS issues among migrants, and UNHCR concentrates mainly on refugees. The scale of their operations is small relative to the needs. The scarcity of resources results in these vulnerable groups being under-served.

Countries in the region lack public understanding of the social and financial costs resulting from increasing HIV/AIDS rates, and consequent potential increase in expensive drug consumption. It is becoming increasingly urgent to raise public awareness. This need cannot be underestimated. For this purpose, a strategic communication plan needs to be implemented at the regional, national and community levels, where the stakeholders are clearly identified, and their interests are addressed. While the public sector does not have capacity to implement a communications strategy, this capacity may exist in the private and academic sectors.

The degree of high-level political commitment differs from country to country. Governments in the region have recognized the need to intervene and avert the epidemic. They have taken several early and appropriate steps to approve appropriate strategies and obtain additional financing, as mentioned before. Nevertheless, political commitment at the level of Head of State and among high-level government officials is still weak. Competing economic and social priorities in these countries overshadow the HIV/AIDS issue in the national debate. The concentration of the epidemic within marginalized groups, who have almost no power to influence public policy making, releases decisionmakers from societal pressures and allows them to partially ignore the issue. Some regional countries try to hide the problem, and as a consequence the health system under-reports HIV. Openness and senior level political discussions about HIV/AIDS, involvement of religious organizations, education of the public about the magnitude of the HIV/AIDS threat to future development, and changing public attitude towards highly vulnerable groups are key actions to be undertaken.

Preventing and controlling the related epidemics requires policy changes such as decriminalization of risk practices, and approval of anti-discrimination laws that require on the one hand know-how, and on the other political will. However, most of the time both are absent because of the stigma attached to highly vulnerable groups; excessive centralization of power; and/or competing priorities. As mentioned before, the existing legislation in most countries is not favorable to marginalized groups. Regional governments are not yet ready to undertake much needed legislative changes. Donor and civil society advocacy is needed to improve the legal rights of the most affected, and to empower vulnerable groups so their voices will be heard by national and sub-national governments.

While all countries have established Country Coordination Mechanisms (CCMs), the effectiveness of these committees is questionable. In reality, National AIDS Centers with assistance from Health Ministries, lead the agenda on control of the HIV/AIDS epidemic.

Interest among different sectors to join the fight against HIV/AIDS has been increasing, but weak collaboration among agencies, and vested interests to control and benefit from donor funding undermine adequate national coordination attempts. Weak government capacity to bring donors around the table and obtain information that is essential for effective planning and adequate resource allocation presents a further challenge.

Although all countries have National HIV/AIDS Committees chaired by Prime Ministers or their deputies, there is an overall lack of leadership and coordination among the different stakeholders. To overcome this weakness, it is necessary that Heads of State become more involved, the National AIDS Committees take more clearly a leadership role; and Drug Control Agencies, and Ministries of Health, Justice and Interior closely cooperate to control the four overlapping epidemics.

Currently, regional collaboration to fight the epidemic is weak. However, these countries have much in common: drug trafficking from Afghanistan through the region, growing numbers of IDUs and CSWs, large-scale regional migration, and human trafficking. National boundaries are weak to prevent the spread of the HIV/AIDS epidemic from one country to the other, and country specific programs combined with a coordinated regional response are necessary to address the epidemic at the regional level.

> **Box 9: The UN Three Ones**
>
> Increasing donor financing creates an opportunity to implement preventive interventions. However, in order to avoid inefficiencies in international funding, it would be necessary to follow the UNAIDS recommendation on the "Three-Ones": one National Strategy, one National Coordinating Mechanism, and one Monitoring and Evaluation system per country.

Additional financial and technical assistance is necessary to overcome institutional weaknesses observed in these countries. UN agencies, GFATM, USAID, DFID, KfW, OSI/Soros Foundation, and others offer assistance to Kazakhstan, the Kyrgyz Republic, Tajikistan, and Uzbekistan to fight HIV/AIDS. Resources available have increased significantly over the last year (Table 10). With assistance from the various donors, initial national capacity to respond to the HIV epidemic has been established. However, due to weak CCMs, donor assistance is inefficient as investments are not well targeted to those most in need. In many cases, donor funding is not accompanied by technical assistance and capacity building activities. Horizontal coordination within national governments and collaboration between various line ministries are weak.

Institutional Capacity to Prevent and Control HIV/AIDS

Preventing and controlling the related epidemics also requires significant institutional changes, such as functional integration of prevention and treatment activities presently undertaken separately by four independent, vertical structures: the Narcology Services, AIDS Centers, Dermatological and Venereal Diseases Dispensaries, and the TB Institutes. However, these structures continue to act independently, with a few examples of good practice—Uzbekistan has already discussed the future overlap between HIV/AIDS and TB—and a few examples of vested interests overtaking the process. Cooperation between the public sector and NGOs, including transfers of funds, is crucial to ensure adequate coverage of highly vulnerable groups. However, this is also hampered by lack of know-how, and/or lack of will. The private sector has not yet been involved in the fight against HIV/AIDS.

Control of the four epidemics also requires adoption of modern, evidence-based practices by groups at risk and professionals. Replacement treatment with methadone or other substitutes of heroin to treat illegal drug use; harm reduction and safe sex approaches for prevention of HIV/AIDS among highly vulnerable groups and vulnerable groups; syndromic treatment of sexually-transmitted infections; and adoption of the WHO-recommended DOTS approach are all being adopted to various degrees by the Central Asia countries. However, there is a need to quickly increase the capacity of these countries to adopt these evidence-based practices, and to appease the resistance to changing practices in some quarters involved in the fight against the epidemics.

In all studied countries, AIDS Centers have assumed a leadership role, with support from MoH. Lab equipment has been purchased, and capacity to carry out testing and diagnosis improved. However, sentinel surveillance is not yet in place, neither monitoring and evaluation systems. The AIDS Centers' ability to work with highly vulnerable groups is limited, as well as the institutional capacity to scale up those interventions as it is necessary. Nevertheless, in all countries there is a strong willingness from these institutions to use funds to offer harm-reduction programs and other preventive services through their infrastructure. These institutions are located in deteriorated facilities with no equipment; they employ underpaid and poorly trained staff; the skill mix is not adequate to offer voluntary testing and counseling, legal assistance and needed preventive and treatment services to highly vulnerable groups. Staff motivation to work with marginalized groups is low. With such institutional weaknesses, adequate implementation of national strategies is at risk.

Local NGOs in these countries have only recently been established. The technical and financial assistance provided by OSI/Soros Foundation, UN agencies and other international partners, helped some NGOs to develop expertise to deal with highly vulnerable groups. However, the number of skilled NGOs is still limited and their geographical coverage is limited to parts of the countries under study. Limited donor funding did not allow them to scale up operations. The quality and modality of services provided by these NGOs is much more acceptable to highly vulnerable groups then those provided by public institutions. Approaches employed are similar to those found in Western countries. Nevertheless, for local NGOs to be able to play a significant role in prevention of the epidemic, more funds and technical assistance are needed to develop their institutional capacity, along with greater influence in policymaking and decisionmaking processes.

International NGOs present in the region include OSI/Soros Foundation,[16] AFEW, and Population Services International (PSI). They have been significantly involved in HIV/AIDS prevention activities in these countries for the past several years, and therefore managed to establish strong collaborative links with Governments, public institutions and civil society.

Routine HIV testing is only now becoming fully available in the Region. Standard HIV surveillance is carried out in testing laboratories located mostly in the AIDS Centers. The samples originate from clinical and population groups as well as blood donations.

---

16. Open Society Institutes are national foundations established in all countries and supported by the Soros Foundation New York.

The extent to which numbers and trends in notified HIV cases reflect the true incidence or prevalence of HIV in the country is limited by both variation in numbers and "case mix" of individuals tested each year. Countries continue to use a system of notification by clinician of clinically confirmed cases of sexually transmitted infection identified through both passive diagnosis in patients requesting clinical services, and through active case finding in sexual contacts of known cases. During the Soviet period this system probably identified the majority of diagnosed cases of syphilis. However, an increasing tendency among patients for self-treatment, a squeeze on funding for STI structures and a lack of availability of reliable diagnostic tests have compromised this approach. Surveillance of drug use and dependency is carried out by the usual system of registration by clinicians working in Narcology Services of clinically confirmed cases of drug use and dependency. Registration rates clearly underestimate the prevalence of drug use in the countries.

With the support of CDC and USAID, Kazakhstan, the Kyrgyz Republic, Tajikistan, and Uzbekistan have been moving towards sentinel surveillance and second-generation surveillance within the framework of "Second Generation HIV Surveillance" recommended by WHO/UNAIDS. Current sites under development include Karaganda, Pavlodar, Uralsk and Shymkent, Bishkek and Osh, Tashkent City, Tashkent Oblast, Andijan, Samarkand and Termis. The focus is on supporting development of laboratory capacity for HIV and hepatitis testing (with some work also on syphilis diagnostics) and quality control systems. Training is being delivered as well as systematic evaluation of the sensitivity and specificity of diagnostics produced in the region. In addition prevalence surveys linked to behavioral surveys are being carried out in risk groups in collaboration with outreach and harm reduction projects. However, additional financial and technical support are necessary to establish appropriate active surveillance throughout the region.

Services for HIV infection in all countries in the Region are delivered through a vertical network of AIDS centers and diagnostic laboratories. These centers provide HIV testing (including screening of predetermined risk groups as well as blood donations), some counseling, treatment for HIV related diseases, as well as carrying out epidemiological interviews with individuals testing positive for HIV. The AIDS Centers also identify areas of, and advocate for critical interventions. All HIV/AIDS Centers have committed themselves to increasing the VCT rates over the coming period as over recent years the number of individuals tested through VCT has been very small. There are continuing problems with supplies of basic medical and laboratory equipment and donor blood is tested inconsistently in all countries. Only palliative treatment is available for those infected with HIV and there is very little use of antiretroviral drugs (ARVs).

Services for both drug users, and STIs are organized in vertical structures with strong traditional links to police and security services. Within drug services, detoxification is almost the only therapeutic treatment offered and engagement with services requires registration. Registration can have serious consequences by de facto excluding the individual from many types of work and leading to loss of employment. It also creates significant difficulties in accessing civic amenities and subsequent dealings with the police. In addition, there may be travel restrictions. Therefore, there are few incentives for individuals to engage with drug services voluntarily, and there is an urgent need to diversify drug services.

STI services are organized along similar lines within the so called "dispensary system." Registration is also required and affordable services can only be obtained in many places with identity documents. Where individuals are infected, they may be rigorously contact traced, in a way that may reveal their condition to friends, associates and communities and entail active police engagement. In addition to the disincentives to testing with registration and its consequences that contact tracing presents, there are serious limitations to both the availability and quality of STI diagnostic tests. This combined with a reluctance on the part of dermato-venereologists to move to syndromic approaches to diagnosis and management, and a strong defense by these specialists of current legal barriers, which prevent other physicians from treating STIs, hinder the shift to delivery of syndromic STI management in primary care, particularly in Kazakhstan and Uzbekistan. This leaves many people who do come to services undiagnosed and untreated.

CHAPTER 3

Reaching a Political and Social Consensus on Timely Implementation of HIV/AIDS Strategies in Central Asia

This study identified the extent of the HIV/AIDS epidemic in Central Asia; developed optimistic and pessimistic scenarios for the potential economic impact of the HIV/AIDS epidemic if early appropriate action is not taken; identified key stakeholders and their roles in preventing and controlling the epidemic; identified gaps in related strategies, policies and legislation; reviewed funding available for prevention and control of HIV/AIDS; and initiated the assessment of the institutional capacity of public services and NGOs to deliver the required services.

Critical gaps were identified that allow this study to make recommendations for key actions that Governments, NGOs, and international partner organizations need to take to ensure timely prevention and control of HIV/AIDS in Central Asia. The study has found that vulnerable groups such as truck drivers and migrants are not presently covered; coverage of highly-vulnerable groups such as injecting drug users (IDUs), commercial sex workers (CSWs) and prisoners is still insignificant; and treatment with anti-retroviral drugs (ARVs) is not yet available in most countries. Additional adequate policies for prevention and treatment need to be adopted; active surveillance (sentinel surveillance and second-generation surveillance) is just beginning with assistance from CDC; and staff and NGOs working in this area need training in evidence-based clinical and public health practices, as well as in program management. These critical gaps, unless addressed promptly, will prevent development of an effective response to the nascent HIV/AIDS epidemic in Central Asia

Reaching a Political and Social Consensus. To address the critical gaps in program implementation it is, however, necessary to reach a wide, multisectoral, political and social consensus regarding the need for early action on HIV/AIDS prevention and control, and to address the regional drivers of the epidemic. While there is some political and social consensus regarding the need to combat drug trafficking and the drug use epidemic—expressed in a Regional Agreement that determined the establishment of Drug Control Agencies throughout the region, and the organization of annual regional meetings to discuss the issue—HIV/AIDS is not yet regarded by policymakers as a priority regional issue, despite the existence of regional and supraregional international agreements. Simultaneously with this Study, Public Opinion Research was carried out in the Kyrgyz Republic (Felzer 2004). Together with the findings of this Study, the POR findings contributed for

---

Reaching a Political and Social Consensus on Timely Implementation of HIV/AIDS Strategies in Central Asia

■ Although early action has been taken in the region to control HIV/AIDS, much remains to be done to ensure proper coverage of highly vulnerable groups and vulnerable groups, and to address the regional drivers of the HIV/AIDS epidemic—drug use and trafficking, human trafficking, and migration.

■ In addition to other activities, advocacy, communication and participation activities have to be undertaken by Governments, NGOs and international organizations to increase the awareness of policymakers, media and the general public about the need to scale up initial actions, as well as to facilitate the participation of various stakeholders—highly-vulnerable groups and vulnerable groups and youth in general, decisionmakers, media, public sector, NGOs and private sector, local and international NGOs and funding organizations—in the decisionmaking process, planning, implementation, and evaluation of key actions.

■ Lessons learned in the region and elsewhere indicate the need for intersectoral action on AIDS, with the involvement of civil society, and the public and private sectors. Effective action requires the involvement in the public sector in Central Asia, of Drug Control Agencies, Ministries of Health, Justice or Interior, Education, and Transport, and Migration Offices. Experience in ECA and elsewhere has shown that when MoHs take the lead, as it has happened with grants from the Global Fund, other sectors (NGOs, private sector, and other ministries) have very limited participation on AIDS prevention activities. For example, prisons, which have the highest number of AIDS cases in the region, have consistently been left out of the early preventive actions, except in Kazakhstan. Therefore, it is necessary to involve Presidential Administrations and Cabinets of Prime Ministers to ensure that all sectors get a fair share of the available resources and take part in the necessary action.

■ Advocacy should be targeted to the highest levels of government, rather than only to the Health Ministry and technical professionals that work exclusively on HIV/AIDS and STIs. Investing in expanding the understanding of policymakers toward best practice, both in and out of the region, will contribute to building the necessary political support that is required to implement the program and underlying reforms.

■ The necessary political support that is required to implement HIV/AIDS programs would increase if policymakers and media had a better understanding of best practices in the region and elsewhere. International partner organizations may want to consider organizing study tours and workshops to inform key decisionmakers and opinionmakers in the different governments about best practices that helped controlling the epidemic in developed countries, and in developing countries such as Brazil and Thailand. The Bank's Global Distance Learning Network (GDLN) will contribute to building of political will and regional capacity.

■ Advocacy and communication activities should be launched to raise public awareness about the needs of highly vulnerable groups, change public attitudes towards them, and to generate public support for the government's policies aimed at combating the HIV/AIDS epidemic. They also need to raise public awareness about the alternative scenarios of the epidemic, adapting data to the peculiarities of priority audiences in each country.

further development of a communication and participation strategy for Central Asia that would aim at improving the existing political and social consensus on timely implementation of HIV/AIDS Strategies in Central Asia. The initial strategy that was designed under this Study is included in Appendix E. In addition, this study has identified other key actions that need to be undertaken to ensure appropriate early action on prevention and control of HIV/AIDS. These are discussed in detail in the box on page 40.

HIV/AIDS Program Coordination. In Central Asia, Deputy Prime Ministers have been chairing AIDS Committees and Country Coordination Mechanisms (CCM). However, the CCMs established to successfully obtain grants from the GFATM, are not functioning in reality as leaders of the fight against the epidemic. All Strategic Plans suggest the need for cross-sectoral collaboration and action. However, in reality, the territoriality of programs is very difficult to overcome. No collaboration exists between Drug Control Agencies, Ministries of Health, Interior, Justice and Education services dealing with the epidemics, and NGOs working with highly vulnerable and vulnerable groups. Weak capacity of the governments to coordinate donor assistance and orchestrate the efforts to combat the epidemic with the help of development partners, puts the current work at risk. The credibility and functionality of the National Coordinating bodies in each country will determine the success of the multi-sectoral activities. Additional efforts are necessary to strengthen coordination mechanisms at the country and regional level. Weak national and regional coordination is just one contributing factor which determines inadequate response.

Strategic and Policy Development. Although these countries have adopted appropriate strategies to fight HIV/AIDS, the detailed analysis of the strategic and legal framework shows that a substantial investment in policy and legislative modernization is needed in each country. Ultimately, the countries will have to decide for themselves how best to change national policy, but the evidence available provides for substantial support for harm reduction and much more extensive substitution therapy. Further policy support for tolerance, human rights protection and appropriate medical and social support for HIV-related medical conditions is needed. In addition, the process of responding to HIV/AIDS

HIV/AIDS Program Coordination

▪ Clear leadership at the highest level of the National AIDS Programs would increase the chances of early prevention of HIV/AIDS in Central Asia. The implementation of National AIDS Programs and of Global Fund grants, and the proposed Regional AIDS Project to be financed by IDA and DFID grants and supported by UNAIDS, would benefit from the direct involvement of Presidents and Prime Ministers of Central Asian countries. The established Country Coordination Mechanisms, which include Governments, NGOs and private sector representatives, should take the strategic lead of the implementation of HIV/AIDS National Programs. Under the leadership of the Country Coordination Mechanisms, intersectoral cooperation between regional Drug Control Agencies, Migration Offices, Narcology Services and AIDS Centers should be promoted and supported.

▪ The establishment of Secretariats for the National Coordination mechanisms would ensure proper functioning of these steering structures. These Secretariats may be financed by the grants available to prevent and control HIV/AIDS in Central Asia.

Strategic and Policy Development

▓ Following up on the approval of National Strategies, regional Governments have started the development of sectoral strategies with assistance from UNAIDS. However, the development of the respective regulatory framework has lagged behind. The legal framework should foster an enabling environment by reducing barriers that contribute to the high incidence of the disease. Program implementation would be facilitated by the adoption of a legal framework in each country that would: (i) protect the rights of people living with HIV/AIDS, including anti-discrimination laws; (ii) facilitate prevention work, such as decriminalization of practices associated with higher risk of HIV/AIDS infection; and (iii) increase access to necessary, confidential medical care, which includes policies on use of anti-retroviral drugs. The legislative and regulatory frameworks should be reviewed to enhance and modify police behavior towards highly vulnerable groups, to reduce criminal management of risk practices and to enhance cross support from health and social agencies for at-risk persons entering the criminal justice system.

▓ Governments have asked the Global Fund to finance treatment of HIV/AIDS with antiretroviral drugs. The regulatory framework should, therefore, include policies on use of antiretroviral drugs following available international evidence and best practices to prevent the advent of drug resistance to ARV.

▓ Countries have now an opportunity to negotiate the prices of antiretroviral drugs to obtain cheaper prices, with assistance from the Bank, GFATM and NGOs such as the Clinton Foundation. This would allow Governments to treat more patients, and ensure the future sustainability of the treatment programs.

▓ Efforts to control HIV/AIDS and STIs should be considered in the context of other ongoing health reform initiatives in Central Asia. Program implementation should address this as an issue of modernizing and improving service delivery. This should build on a 'how-to-get-things done' approach, and would include preventive, diagnostic, treatment and rehabilitation services. Some degree of integration between Narcology Services, STIs Dispensaries, TB Institutes and AIDS Centers would be desirable to address the overlap between the epidemics of drug use, STIs, HIV/AIDS and TB; and to increase efficiency and effectiveness. Salaries and benefit packages of public health staff should be reviewed to provide proper incentives and focus.

▓ Review of the legal and financial basis and mechanisms for contractual relationships between Government and NGOs should be carried out to deliver a simpler framework that facilitates the establishment of effective partnerships between the public sector and NGOs.

---

has been isolated from the broader thrust of health sector reform. Government and grant funding, especially from the GFATM, continue to reinforce existing vertical structures, which will not contribute to a sustainable solution; and key elements of comprehensive programs including expanding availability and modernization of STI Services and Narcology Services are in some cases being actively blocked by relevant professional groups.

Surveillance and Monitoring and Evaluation. Central Asia countries have been upgrading the surveillance system with assistance from CDC and funding from USAID. However, this key activity requires further support. No reliable HIV surveillance data are available, and attempts to estimate prevalence among highly vulnerable groups (IDUs, CSWs, prisoners) have been confounded by technical difficulties. Monitoring and evaluation capacity remains weak. On monitoring and evaluation, the lack of early response systems based on monitoring inputs and outputs has weakened the early efforts to implement

---

Surveillance and Monitoring and Evaluation

- The ongoing regional program to improve sentinel and second generation surveillance of HIV/AIDS with assistance from USAID/CDC should be further supported, technically and financially, by Governments and international donors. Second generation surveillance should cover new geographical areas and risk groups through harm reduction and outreach programs, including Trust Points. The identification of highly-vulnerable groups and vulnerable groups by the public sector and NGOs, with assistance from international organizations, should continue, including estimates of their size that provide denominators that allow to determine incidence and prevalence rates.

- Laboratory infrastructure will continue to be improved with assistance from USAID and KfW. In addition to HIV and hepatitis testing, this should include establishment of STI reference laboratories.

- The UN-recommended principle of one M&E system per country should be followed, which requires coordination among different stakeholders financing and implementing programs. This coordination should be undertaken in the context of the CCM. Clear indicators of success may be prepared by AIDS Centers in consultation with others stakeholders, and should be agreed by CCMs. These indicators would track epidemiological data, behavioral data and regional drivers of the epidemic. Capacity to analyze data needs to be further developed.

- The proposed Regional AIDS Project will complement ongoing efforts to establish regional second generation surveillance, and to establish an integrated regional Monitoring and Evaluation system.

GFTAM grants. Furthermore, there are few impact assessments of the efforts by international organizations to fight the epidemic.

Capacity Building. Capacity building activities have been undertaken, especially with assistance from CDC in the area of second generation surveillance. However, this is an area that requires additional investment. Lack of capacity (institutional and technical) among state institutions and local NGOs, who have to play a critical role in reaching out high-risk groups, is one of the factors that limits the implementation of agreed strategies. The institutional assessment confirms significant deficiencies (structural and regarding human resources) within health care systems, which prevents them from offering the needed diagnostic, preventive and curative services to high-risk groups. Prevention efforts have almost exclusively taken a pilot site approach led by international organizations and NGOs. As a result of this, the implementation capacity of the country-based agencies has not been adequately considered or reinforced. This is particularly true in relation to the Governments' ability to implement policy; and to procure and contract activities from NGOs. These problems are already undermining the implementation of Global Fund grants in several countries (Kazakhstan and the Kyrgyz Republic, as it has happened in Ukraine) and will potentially limit the cost-effectiveness, and even existence of these and other grant-funded programs.

The number of local NGOs in the Central Asian region that work with high risk groups and provide critical services/intervention for the control of the epidemic, has been rapidly increasing. However, current coverage of at risk groups by these organizations is largely inadequate and calls for additional technical and financial assistance for capacity building. Finally, there is little involvement of the private sector and communities in prevention and

---

Capacity Building

▓ Training of public services and NGOs has been provided on a limited scale. This is an area in which the proposed Regional AIDS Project may make a significant contribution to building regional capacity to tackle the HIV/AIDS epidemic.

▓ Public Health skills and capacity need to be increased at all levels through: (i) training existing staff and (ii) providing additional incentives for them. Training programs have to reach out medical professionals, local NGOs, community organizations, prison, police and border control staff, and tourism workers.

▓ Capacity building for NGOs is a critical activity that will promote long-term sustainability of the programs and improve implementation. Programs launched by Governments and international partners should provide: (i) technical assistance for training prior to launching activities; (ii) resources to link NGOs with information technology and connectivity that will enhance their performance; (iii) strong monitoring and evaluation of the NGO performance; and (iv) consider elements of sustainability from the beginning. The public sector should be trained in contracting NGOs to implement activities, which should be delivered at national and local government levels.

▓ Local NGOs, not international NGOs, should play a predominant role in the HIV/AIDS program's implementation. They should be clearly identified and targeted as the distribution channel for many of the programs. The success of Brazil's program, for example, is largely built on the work of local NGOs. Support should be provided for NGO development in geographical areas where service provision is lacking or is absent; and/or enhance the capacity of existing ones to scale up their operations to those regions.

▓ Efforts should be made to build public-private partnerships. This includes expanding the role of the private sector to introduce prevention activities and IEC at the workplace, but also using the private sector to extend access to basic commodities (condoms, syringes, gel and drugs) and to advocate for HIV/AIDS issues at Government level.

▓ Municipalities should be actively involved in the prevention of the drug use and HIV/AIDS epidemics. Mobilize communities to participate in promotion and prevention efforts, tapping into the existing cultural, private and faith-based organizations to secure a sustained, caring and effective outreach service. Strategic communications at the community level will solicit the mobilization of group resources, generating responses in tune with prevailing values and beliefs, and increasing sustainability and effectiveness.

---

control of HIV/AIDS, although the potential for this may be considerable due to the existence in the region of oil, mining, food, tourism and other important industries.

Regional Drivers and Coverage of Highly-vulnerable Groups. There have been limited efforts to address the regional threats, or future drivers, of the epidemic. These include, among others: drug-trafficking and use, migration and trafficking of women. Coverage of highly vulnerable groups (IDUs, CSWs, prisoners, youth at risk) is still well below desirable targets. In addition, vulnerable groups such as migrants and truck drivers also need to be covered to prevent a major epidemic. For example, in the Kyrgyz Republic, about 60 percent of youth will be covered by information, education and communication (IEC) activities, but less than 30 percent of highly vulnerable groups, and only 5 percent of IDUs will be reached by harm reduction activities, which are those that can most contribute to preventing the spread of the infection. Gaps in coverage are partly due to insufficiency of funding and partly due to lack of coordination among the different stakeholders.

Regional Drivers and Coverage of Highly-vulnerable Groups

- Injecting drug users and commercial sex workers, along with prisoners, are currently the groups most at risk and, therefore, the most risky channel for HIV transmission. Preventing the spread of HIV among these groups is advisable to prevent subsequent sexual transmission to vulnerable groups that do not inject drugs, and/or are not partners of drug users.

- Partnerships between Governments, NGOs and international organizations have allowed initial coverage of groups most at risk. These partnerships should be pursued to ensure scaling-up of prevention programs, especially among highly vulnerable groups to reach a proportion of these (50–60 percent) that enables adequate control of the epidemic.

- The ongoing regional cooperation to prevent drug trafficking and drug use should be further supported by UNODC and other agencies.

- The proposed Regional AIDS Control Project will specifically focus on regional drivers of the epidemics of drug use, sexually-transmitted diseases, HIV/AIDS and TB. Resources will be focused on epidemiological hotspots where sentinel surveillance suggests that the observed regional differences in notification are not artefactual. The results of the mapping study have informed the preparation of the Regional AIDS Project, which will give priority to developing processes, structures and networks that promote and facilitate lesson learning and experience sharing across the region at all levels.

Funding of HIV/AIDS Programs. This study suggests that significant gaps in funding of HIV/AIDS programs persist: on the one hand, less than 25 percent of groups at risk will be covered with available funding, including funding from the GFATM; on the other hand, according to initial estimates, available funding is a small proportion of funding needs if best practices on prevention and control are followed. While GFATM grants have become available, and funding from Governments, international agencies, and bilateral agencies has been increasing, funds are insufficient to finance critical interventions or are used inefficiently due to lack of coordination between Governments and donors, and among donors. Additional financial resources need to be put in place to deliver interventions at a scale necessary to have an epidemiological impact; support national and regional coordination; strengthen institutional capacity of national agencies and local NGOs; and further develop adequate technical expertise so much needed in the region as a whole and in each country.

Funding of HIV/AIDS Programs

- Coordination of different stakeholders, under the leadership of the Country Coordination Mechanisms (CCMs), would improve the efficiency and effectiveness of fund use.

- Governments should increase budget allocations and raise additional funding for prevention and control of HIV/AIDS. Funding should be raised to enable increased coverage, and more efficient use should be made of existing resources.

- There must be significant investment in policy development, management and coordination capacity especially focused on the management of GFATM and other grants; fund disbursement by Governments to NGOs; and overcoming structural political and vested interests barriers to implementation.

- The proposed Regional AIDS Control project will not only contribute additional resources to enable civil society and regional Governments to tackle the epidemic, but will also establish a mechanism for sustainable management of available grant funding.

The World Bank's Role: Regional AIDS Control Project

The World Bank will continue to assist the Region's Governments in overcoming some of the identified critical gaps in four different ways:

- ▓ by pursuing advocacy and policy dialogue conducive to increasing political will to take early action to prevent and control the four overlapping epidemics;
- ▓ by carrying out further sector work that will increase the understanding about the four related epidemics;
- ▓ by assisting the implementation of a proposed Regional AIDS Control Project that will contribute to decreasing the potential negative impact of a major HIV/AIDS epidemic on regional development; and
- ▓ by providing technical and financial support at country level for implementation of the national programs aimed at controlling the four epidemics.

During the last two years, stakeholder workshops have been organized to learn more about clients' demand for TB and HIV/AIDS activities, and to build consensus regarding early adoption of appropriate strategies to fight HIV/AIDS and the Bank's role in this area. The *Central Asia HIV/AIDS and TB Country Profiles* were discussed with stakeholders, and distributed in the region and among international partner organizations. The *Central Asia AIDS Study* and other regional studies undertaken by the Bank in this area were also reviewed by regional stakeholders. The Bank will organize further advocacy and learning activities through GDLN.

In November 2003, following initial sector work, the Bank and DFID started discussions with Governments of Central Asia about the possibility of financing a Regional AIDS Project that would further assist implementation of the regional strategy to control HIV/AIDS. Project Identification Workshops following a logical framework approach took place in Kazakhstan, Kyrgyz Republic, Tajikistan, and Uzbekistan. Representatives from Ministries of Health, Interior, Justice, Education, Labor and Social Protection, Drug Control Agencies, among others, actively participated in these workshops. In addition, local and international NGOs and partner organizations have been consulted regarding project design and implementation.

In the context of project preparation, the Governments of Kazakhstan, Kyrgyz Republic, Tajikistan, and Uzbekistan have been showing commitment to prevention and control of HIV/AIDS in Central Asia. In June 2004, Deputy Prime Ministers signed a Memorandum of Understanding at a high-level meeting organized by UNAIDS, DFID, and the World Bank in Almaty, commiting to cooperate on the preparation of the Regional AIDS Project, The Central Asia Cooperation Agreement, which will provide the legal framework for project implementation, has been ratified by participating countries. Senior staff of several Ministries, NGOs and private sector representatives from these countries have participated in three Regional Technical Meetings for project preparation; and high-level delegations from the four countries participated in the project negotiations. The Project is expected to become effective in July 2005.

A regional operation will have several advantages:

- ▓ First, major epidemic drivers act regionally and can therefore best be addressed at a regional level. These include: trafficking of people and drugs, economic and political migration, and commercial sex work;

- Second, constraints upon developing an effective response are common in all countries in the region as are the tools to overcome these. These include: advocacy and communication needs, legislative and regulatory reform, improving surveillance and use of data for decisionmaking, approaches to managing professional resistance to change, and changing police behavior;
- Third, there is a need to deliver economies of scale in terms of both financial and human resources, through developing regional activities in key areas. These include: training programs for capacity building in all aspects of response design and delivery; development of best practice guidelines and protocols in relation to training and policy design processes; commissioning activities, PPP, and sentinel surveillance; STI, IDU and HIV management protocols; and improving delivery of ART;
- Finally, there is great capacity for transferring experience from countries which have solved problems to those which have not at both macro and micro level in relation to harm reduction, modernization of services, and NGO development.

The Project includes a Policy Development and Institutional Capacity Building Component and a Regional AIDS Fund. The first component will assist Governments with further regulatory development, and building of surveillance and institutional capacity. The second component will contribute to: (i) increase coverage of highly vulnerable groups; (ii) increase participation of civil society, public and private sectors in HIV/AIDS control in Central Asia; and (iii) developing partnerships among different sectors and agencies. The Fund will finance public and private agencies, and NGOs working with highly vulnerable and vulnerable groups along the regional corridors (the Northern Corridor and the Silk Route) used for transporting people (CSWs, trafficked people, refugees, labor migrants, traders, truck drivers, travel, customs and law enforcement staff, etc) and goods (especially drugs). It will also fund agencies working with risk groups in the prison system. Project preparation activities are under way which will improve knowledge of how the epidemic is evolving; continue to trace the regional drivers of the epidemic; and improve the availability of information required for advocacy and further policy development.

APPENDIXES

Epidemiological and Programmatic Update

Key Findings in Kazakhstan

There has been a five-fold increase in registered IDUs since the beginning of the 1990s. Estimates of a total number of drug users of around 200,000 (1.25 per 100,000) are constant in all available data. In 2004, 699 new cases of HIV positive were identified in the country, bringing the cumulative number to 4,696 (31.4 per 100,000) by the end of 2004, of which three quarters are IDUs. Current Government estimates put the number of persons living with HIV in Kazakhstan at more than 25,000, with over 80 percent of HIV-positive persons believed to be drug users. Syphilis incidence increased from 1.5 per 100,000 in 1990, to 231 per 100,000 in 1996, but then decreased to stabilize around 109 per 100,000 in 2002. It is not clear to what extent the decline in syphilis notifications since the mid-1990s reflects a true decrease in incidence or a decline in the number of people who turn to official medical services. There are strong indications that the most vulnerable groups—IDUs, CSWs, MSMs, migrants, and prisoners—have seen rapid increases in the country over the recent years. There are an estimated 200,000 IDUs and 20,000 CSWs in the country and levels of risk behavior appear to be high.

Strategic plans call for an inter-sectoral approach and this appears to have been achieved at high governmental level. In 2002, inter-sectoral strategic AIDS response programs for the period up to 2005 were developed by the Ministries of Health, Education, Defense, Interior, Justice, Culture, and Information. AIDS Coordination Committees were established at the ministries to implement strategic AIDS prevention and control programs. The Republican AIDS Center with technical and financial support from UNAIDS and other UN agencies, played a major role in this process, but the input of NGOs in the process, and indeed the role of NGOs more broadly in the field, is weak. The CCM, which was formed for Global Fund grant application and implementation, successfully applied

Kazakhstan: Key Indicators at a Glance (2004)	
AIDS/HIV Deaths	159
AIDS Cases—Cumulative	64
AIDS Cases—New	231
	78
HIV Cases—Cumulative	4,696
HIV Cases—Cum/100,000	31.4
M:F Ratio HIV—Cumulative	3:1 (men—3,597; women—1,099)
Proportion of HIV Cumulative among 20–29 years old	54% (2,531 cases)
HIV Cumulative among IDU	3,640 cases (77.5%)
HIV Cases—New	699
Proportion of New HIV among IDU	62% (433 cases)
HIV Cases—New/100,000	4.7
M:F Ratio New Cases	2:1
Oblast w/highest new HIV rate	Almaty city
New HIV /100,000 (all ages) in Almaty City	17 (48.4 cumulative)
Estimated HIV Prevalence IDU	3.2%
Estimated HIV Prevalence Prisoners (males)	0.7%
Estimated prevalence in pregnant women	0.1%
Registered Drug Users	
M:F Sex Ratio Drug Users	7:1
Registered IDU	34,374
Estimated IDU	200–250,000
Estimated HIV Preval. IDU	3.2% < 5%
Estimated CSW	20,000
Estimated MSM	31,800

for grants for HIV/AIDS and TB, and meets on a regular basis. However, some institutions are concerned that the MoH does not have a strong interest in the HIV/AIDS program and does not provide adequate funding. There are serious concerns among UN agencies and within some of the state bodies that resistance among narcologists and dermato-venereal disease specialists to some of the innovations planned within the GFATM program will make delivery extremely difficult. The Government of Kazakhstan has recognized the need to intervene to avert the epidemic, has put in place coherent strategies, and has secured funds through international donors and the GFATM. However, significant barriers remain to delivering a timely response.

Surveillance for drug use, HIV/AIDS and STIs continue to depend on compulsory notification/registration systems and outdated screening programs, which persist from the Soviet era. The validity of the findings from these systems, as to whether notification rates and trends reflect the true underlying incidence and prevalence of these diseases or the distribution of risk among clinical, population or GOR, is likely to continue to decline.

CDC is developing a network of quality control laboratories (primarily testing for HIV and hepatitis markers) and linking these to prevalence and behavioral surveys among risk groups. There is an urgent need to ensure that sentinel and second-generation surveillance approaches continue to be supported and extended as new waves of harm reduction and prevention projects reach new geographic locations and risk sub groups. There is currently no sentinel surveillance for STIs.

HIV/AIDS and STIs in Kazakhstan: Epidemiological Trends

Drug Use. The number and rates of currently registered drug users are shown in Figure 2. The figure shows a five-fold increase in registered IDUs since the beginning of the 1990s, although the rate of increase has declined, stabilizing between 2002 and 2003. UNODC has estimated that 25 percent of drug users in the country are registered. If this is the case, then the total number of drug users would be around 200,000 (1.25 per 100,000).

HIV/AIDS. Current Government estimates put the number of persons living with HIV in Kazakhstan at more than 25,000; with over 80 percent of HIV-positive persons estimated to be drug users. Figure 3 shows new and cumulative notifications and notification rates per 100,000. Cumulative cases increased rapidly from 1996 to reach 4001 (23.9 per 100,000) by the end of 2003. New cases identified have varied with the number of tests performed and groups tested but have stabilized around 700 per year (4.5 per 100,000) over the last 2 years.

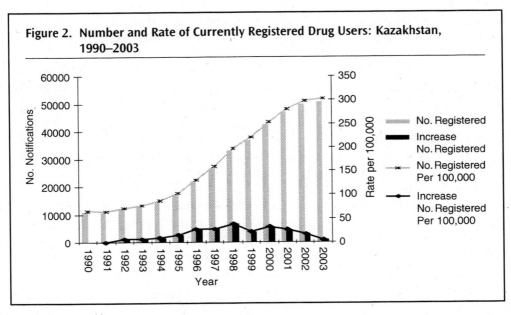

Figure 2. Number and Rate of Currently Registered Drug Users: Kazakhstan, 1990–2003

Source: MoH Kazakhstan.

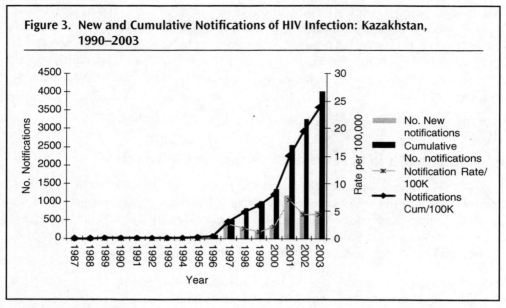

Figure 3. New and Cumulative Notifications of HIV Infection: Kazakhstan, 1990–2003

Source: MoH Kazakhstan.

Figure 4 shows the age distribution of cases in each year since 1997. In 2002, 20,437 injecting drug users were tested for HIV infection, and of these, 217 were found to be positive. The peak age group is aged 20–29 for all years since 1997, with around half of all cases consistently falling into this age group. Cumulative rates among 20–29 year-olds approach 0.1 percent of the population, and rates among 15–19 year-olds and 30–39 year-olds are similar. In the same year 22,400 pregnant women were tested for HIV infection, of which 76 were found to be positive.

According to the Kazakh AIDS Center, the epidemiological "hotspots" in the country are: Karaganda, Pavlodar, South Kazakhstan, and Kostanai Oblasts, and the city of Almaty. Figure 5 shows the regional and sex distribution of new cases of HIV infection in Kazakhstan for 2001. The figure shows a concentration of notifications in that year in Pavlodar, which may reflect numbers of tests carried out there. However, it is remarkable that the notification rate exceeded 0.1 percent among males in that year. It may be inferred that the notification rate among males reached 0.5 percent of men in that age group in that year.

The number of HIV tests carried out in Kazakh prisons and the number of HIV positive cases by age and sex are shown in Table 11. This table shows prevalence rates close to 0.1 percent among men and women tested in 2001. Prevalence rates among men and women were lower in 2002, but this may reflect a different testing policy in prisons as testing became voluntary, and with testing moving out to lower risk subgroups. Provisional results of sentinel surveillance of people attending voluntary testing and counseling suggest HIV prevalence rates of 5 percent in Karaganda, 2 percent in Uralsk and 0.3 percent in Almaty.

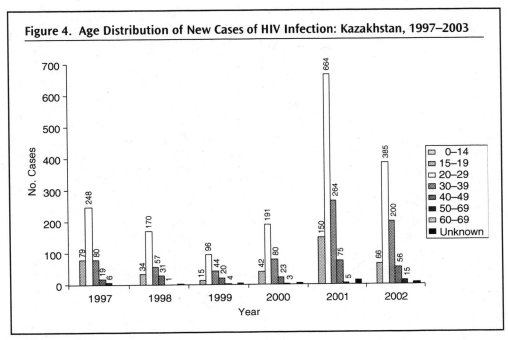

Figure 4. Age Distribution of New Cases of HIV Infection: Kazakhstan, 1997–2003

Source: MoH Kazakhstan.

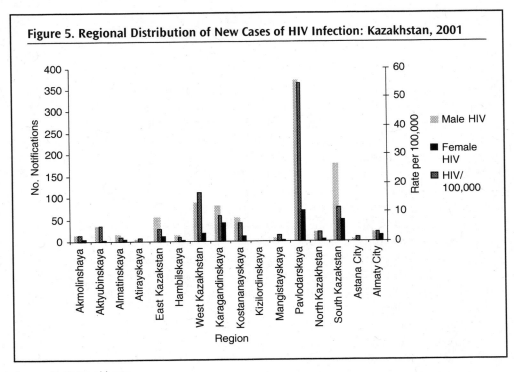

Figure 5. Regional Distribution of New Cases of HIV Infection: Kazakhstan, 2001

Source: MoH Kazakhstan.

Table 11. Number of HIV Tests Carried Out in Prisons and HIV Cases by Age and Sex: Kazakhstan: 1999–2002

Year	Age	Men Tested	No. Men HIV+	Men Rate per 100,000	Women Tested	No. Women HIV+	Women Rate per 100,000
1999	All ages	73872	2	3	3801	0	0
2000	All ages	74623	7	9	3685	0	0
2001	All ages	41948	40	95	3756	3	80
2002	All ages	67265	17	25	3353	1	30
2002	15–24	3658	0	0	189	0	0
2002	25–34	35014	12	34	1245	1	80
2002	35–44	27373	3	11	1008	0	0
2002	45–54	1112	2	180	715	0	0
2002	55–64	108	0	0	196	0	0

Source: MoH Kazakhstan.

STI. No information on numbers or rates of syphilis or other STI notifications were made available by the Ministry of Health of Kazakhstan so far. However, previously published information suggests, as mentioned in the summary, that the syphilis incidence rate increased from 1.5 per 100,000 in 1990 to 231 per 100,000 in 1996, but then stabilized around 109 per 100,000 in 2002. Thus, the size of the epidemic has been large in Kazakhstan.

Risk Behavior and Environment

The Kazakh economy experienced a period of steep economic decline during the 1990s, but grew 13.5 percent in 2001 with higher oil prices and increased oil and gas production in the country, with GNP reaching $1,510 in 2002 (Asian Development Bank 2001). USAID (2003) estimated that the unemployment rate in 2002 might have been as high as 30 percent, while, according to the UNDP report (2003), over 30 percent of population was living in poverty at the end of the 1990s. Since the Soviet period, educational opportunities for young people have been reduced and there has been a serious deterioration in social services (Human Rights Watch 2003). At the same time, there has been an explosion in injecting drug use and commercial sex work with the development of local markets for opiates that has been trafficked from Afghanistan since the early 1990s. This explosion, combined with the simultaneous STI epidemic and economic migration, including shuttle migration to high HIV prevalence areas in the CIS and elsewhere, have created a serious threat of a major HIV epidemic, initially concentrated among IDUs, but with potential to rapidly generalize through sexual transmission.

Globally, the most vulnerable groups for HIV infection are IDUs, CSWs, MSM, migrants, and prisoners. Anecdotal data and rapid assessments suggest that the last 14 years have seen rapid increases in size of these groups in Kazakhstan (UNAIDS 2002c). These changes, together with high levels of risk behavior, are driven by increased income differentials and poverty, the passage of drug trafficking routes carrying opiates through the country, and hostile and dishonest police behavior in relation to highly vulnerable groups. High levels of migration, including to destinations with higher background prevalence of HIV infection such as Russia, are likely to be continuously seeding infection into the population. Decline in social support services and participation in education as well as high unemployment leave young people increasingly vulnerable to risk behaviors associated with HIV infection. Public attitudes to people infected with HIV continue to be highly stigmatizing. Levels of awareness about the infection, modes of its transmission, and ways of protection from it are still low. The Government of Kazakhstan has been working to improve the legislative and policy frameworks through modifying the testing strategy for HIV, ending segregation of HIV-positive prisoners, and reviewing HIV/AIDS- related regulations and laws.

Increasing income differentials and poverty create demand for and supply of CSW, while the passage of drug trafficking routes carrying opiates through the country delivers a copious supply of cheap opium and heroin to fuel the epidemic of injecting drug use. Hostile and dishonest police behavior in relation to CSW and IDU is widespread in the country; and such behavior is known to be a key factor driving CSW and IDU into patterns of behavior associated with very high risk of HIV transmission (Human Rights Watch 2003). High levels of migration, including to destinations with higher background prevalence of HIV infection such as Russia, are likely to be continuously seeding infection into the population as well as leaving young women alone at home and unsupported and vulnerable. A decline in social support services and participation in education as well as unemployment leaves young people increasingly vulnerable to HIV risk behaviors and infection.

Levels of awareness of HIV, modes of transmission and ways of protection are higher than in other countries of the region. A public opinion survey was undertaken in 2004 to assess public awareness, attitudes and practices vis-à-vis HIV/AIDS.[17] About half of those interviewed were aware of the disease and 30 percent had a detailed knowledge; two thirds were aware of ways of transmission; however, only 16 percent correctly identified all sources of HIV infection. These results showed that the population needs to know more about voluntary testing and prevention of HIV/AIDS. In addition, less than half (46 percent) of the interviewed rejected the need to isolate HIV/AIDS patients, which suggests that much remains to be done in what concerns stigma and discrimination.

The Government of Kazakhstan has taken several positive steps recently. In 2002, it lifted the national policy of mandatory HIV testing for a wide range of groups, including drug users and those in pre-trial detention. It has also announced an end to the policy of segregating HIV-positive prisoners. A revision of HIV/AIDS relevant regulations and laws is being undertaken to bring them into line with international standards on HIV/AIDS and human rights.

The number of registered drug users has stabilized. Triangulated evidence points to around 200,000 or more drug users in the country, of which perhaps 180,000 are injecting drug users. There is evidence of high levels of risk behavior including sharing of injecting

---

17. The survey was carried out in the context of the GFATM grant (see AIDS Center 2004).

equipment (Human Rights Watch 2003). Rates of injecting drug use are far higher among men, but it is likely that those among women are less accurately estimated in routine data gathering. Drug users are becoming younger and there are reports of a shift away from traditional opium injection to heroin injection (WHO Information Centre on Health for CAR 2003). This may have benefits as well as disadvantages in relation to HIV transmission. The extent to which female injecting drug users engage in commercial sex work to earn money to purchase drugs is unknown. Surveys carried out by UNAIDS suggest that there is awareness among IDUs of HIV risks: 88 percent know that disposable syringes protect from HIV infection and 95 percent know that condoms can prevent HIV transmission. Despite this, risk behavior continues to be pervasive (Godinho and others 2004).

According to 2002 sentinel surveillance data, 13.5 percent of IDUs engage in commercial sex work to obtain money or drugs. The number of CSWs in the country is unknown; however some Government and international agency sources estimate this to be as high as 20–50,000 (Godinho 2004). A systematic attempt to estimate the number of CSWs in Almaty in 1996 suggested that there were 2,500 CSWs working in the city (Thomas 1996). It was reported in Almaty in 2000, that 70 percent of CSWs previously had STI (Zhusupov 2000). More recently, HIV prevalence surveys among CSWs in the country showed that 0.5 percent out of 4,000 people surveyed were HIV infected (Gotsadze 2003). The Government's application to the GFATM suggests that over half of CSWs do not use condoms, and that 10–30 percent may provide sex in exchange for drugs.

There is still very little information concerning the number of or risk behavior among men having sex with men (MSM). One survey (Gotsadze 2003) conducted in Almaty city in 2003 suggests that condoms are used by MSM in only 20 percent of cases, and there are substantial rates of STIs (25 percent) and drug use (10 percent) in this group.

Prevention and Control

The strategic framework and stakeholder action are analyzed in detail elsewhere in this report.

Surveillance. Surveillance of drug use and dependency is carried out by a system of registration of clinically confirmed cases by clinicians working in Narcology Services. There is a statutory obligation for physicians to maintain newly identified individuals on this register until they meet formal criteria for removal. Registration rates clearly underestimate the prevalence of drug use in the country, but UNODC (2003) estimates that as many as 25 percent of all drug users may be registered.

Routine HIV surveillance is carried out through health service structures in testing laboratories located mostly in the AIDS centers. The samples originate from clinical and population groups and blood donations. Tested groups include: registered drug users, patients with STI diagnoses, and pregnant women. Testing is irregular; it varies in particular with test availability. Positive screening tests are required to be confirmed by the Western Blot. Persons identified as being HIV infected are invited to attend clinical services where an epidemiological interview is conducted to establish key demographic variables and likely route of transmission. Information on HIV positive individuals is completed and put in standard notification forms and statistical summaries that are then sent down to the Center.

The extent to which numbers and trends in notified cases reflect the true incidence or prevalence of HIV in the country is limited by both variation in number and "case mix" of individuals tested each year. Kazakhstan continues to use a system of notification by a clinician of clinically confirmed cases of STIs as the primary means of STI surveillance. There is a statutory obligation for physicians to notify each person who is newly identified as being infected with a sexually transmitted disease the notification of which is mandatory (syphilis and gonorrhea). Infected individuals are identified through both passive diagnosis in patients seeking clinical services and active case-findings of previous sexual contacts of detected cases. During the Soviet period this system probably identified the majority of diagnosed cases of syphilis. However, since 1990 it is highly likely that there has been a decline in accuracy of notifications as a result of: (i) an increasing tendency among patients to use paid anonymous services obtained in public or private clinics; (ii) lack of funding for the Dermato-Venereal Diseases and STI structures; and (iii) lack of availability of sensitive and specific diagnostic tests and strict case definitions for reporting, which do not reflect the fact that cases may be syndromically diagnosed and managed.

With the support of CDC, USAID, and UNAIDS, the country is moving towards adoption of sentinel surveillance within the framework of the Second-Generation HIV Surveillance recommended by WHO/UNAIDS (2000). In 2003, pilot sentinel sites were established in Karaganda, Pavlodar, South Kazakhstan and West Kazakhstan. In 2004, sentinel surveillance was extended to six regions: Kostanai, East Kazakhstan, Akmola, North Kazakhstan oblasts, and the cities of Astana and Almaty. It is expected that the entire country will be covered by sentinel surveillance sites in 2005. The focus is on supporting development of laboratory capacity for HIV and hepatitis testing, with some work also done on syphilis diagnostics and quality control systems. Training as well as systematic evaluation of the sensitivity and specificity of diagnostics produced in the region are being carried out. In addition, prevalence surveys linked to behavioral surveys are being conducted among risk groups in collaboration with outreach and harm-reduction projects.

Surveillance of STIs is similar to that in other CA countries, and the technical base of this service has also declined significantly over the last 10 years due to decreasing Government funding. Reliable syphilis diagnosis is available in urban centers but there are no reliable tests available for chlamydia infection or for gonorrhea infection in women. Availability of essential STI drugs may be good but needs to reviewed, and there are reports of shortages in the periphery. Patients pay for all treatments. Substantial number of patients appears still to be managed as inpatients. Progress with modernization of STI services through their delivery within primary care structures, or through using syndromic management approaches in the absence of available laboratory diagnostic facilities has proved difficult to achieve. Practices in relation to contact tracing may still follow old Soviet models. The dermato-venereal service has found it difficult to adapt to new circumstances and accept innovations. There is an urgent need to find ways to move STI service delivery forward and to remove obstacles to innovation and development that are presented by medical professionals. There is currently a need for strong political support for implementation of syndromic diagnosis and management of STIs and adaptation of protocols to local epidemiological and infrastructure conditions. It is especially important to persuade the medical establishment that syndromic management is "scientific" and justified.

Prevention among Vulnerable Groups. The President of Kazakhstan has commissioned a study to consider the legalization of cannabis and hashish and reduced penalties for drug users as part of "humanizing" their treatment. The structure of the Narcology Services still follows the old Soviet system, with a country wide network of Narcology Dispensaries including inpatient facilities for detoxification. There is considerable resistance among narcologists to methadone substitution therapy. However, two pilot methadone substitution therapy programs started operating in 2003.

A system of 98 "Trust Points" has been established by the Government to provide services to IDUs and other marginalized groups, aiming to provide harm reduction commodities and information. These are usually located in outpatient clinics, but there are plans to use other venues as well. There are, however, anecdotal reports of significant problems with the functioning of these points including: police harassment of attendees, lack of commodities, and lack of confidence among the vulnerable groups in their confidentiality. There is a need for training that would increase the skills and capacity of the largely volunteer staff of these trust points. The Soros Foundation/Open Society Institute (OSI) is closing its drug harm reduction program. A new program focusing on drug demand reduction is currently being implemented under OSI management, but this will not focus on harm reduction or needle exchange.

Traditionally, little emphasis has been placed on the primary prevention of STIs through education and health promotion initiatives, although case-finding and contact-tracing have been assiduously carried out. There is increased provision of health promotion materials in some STI clinics. However, condoms are not currently offered at these clinics, either for free or even for a fee.

Clinical and Laboratory Services. Clinical and laboratory services are provided through the network of over 21 territorial AIDS Centers throughout the country. Recent technical inputs from CDC have strengthened the quality of laboratory work, but availability of antiretroviral therapy for HV/AIDS is still severely limited. Voluntary counseling and testing (VCT) is available in some areas but is not widely or consistently implemented.

A total of 977 dermato-venereal disease specialists are registered in Kazakhstan. Prior to the break-up of the Former Soviet Union, the old Soviet system operated in full, and it still forms the basis of the current public sector system for control of STIs in Kazakhstan. The services comprised diagnostic, treatment and contact-tracing facilities backed up by legal powers to force those found to be infected to undergo treatment and to identify their previous sexual contacts. Individuals were required to produce identity papers in order to be examined in these facilities. Infected individuals were prevented from accessing a variety of municipal facilities, certain types of work and travel until certified as having been cured. There were minimum requirements for their success in tracing "sources" of infection.

Over recent years, although the old structures are still in place, it has become clear that many people now seek advice and treatment for sexually transmitted diseases outside the public sector. Some attend private physicians, while others self-treat infections in order to avoid the stigma and coercion embedded in the public system. The diagnosis, treatment and contact tracing offered within private settings may be carried out by physicians with no specialized training in STIs. It is believed that it is now possible to obtain anonymous diagnosis and treatment within the public system, but the service would be paid under the table.

The approach to diagnosis and management of STIs remains based on etiological diagnosis, although there is anecdotal evidence that the availability of high quality laboratory diagnostics within the public system has declined significantly over recent years. There were reports of very strong political resistance among members of the public establishment to the introduction of syndromic STI management and that this was derailing implementation of proposed shift to the new system envisioned under the implementation of the GFATM grant. Zdrav plus, with support from USAID, has run pilots integrating syndromic diagnosis and management into primary care delivery structures with considerable success. The main barriers to success have been considerable additional workload it has created for primary care staff and their reluctance to add work on a long-term basis without additional compensation.

Key Findings in the Kyrgyz Republic

About 6,000 drug users are registered in the country, but it is estimated that the real number is much higher, and that there are about 70,000 IDUs. In 2003, 132 new cases of HIV were identified in the country, bringing the cumulative number to 508, of which 421 are IDUs. Annual numbers of notified cases of syphilis increased from 2 per 100,000 in 1990 to 167 per 100,000 in 1997, but then declined and stabilized around 50 per 100,000 by 2002.

The Government of the Kyrgyz Republic has been active in grasping the significance of the HIV and sexually transmitted disease epidemics for the country. Although the central Government commitment to fight HIV/AIDS is in place, further advocacy is necessary to engage the Presidential Administration and national Government in the control of the epidemic. The Strategic Plan to control HIV/AIDS epidemic in the country was developed through a broad Government and NGO consultation process. Most NGOs specializing in work with CSWs, IDUs, MSM and other highly vulnerable groups contributed to the development of this strategy along with public institutions. Despite strong ownership, significant barriers remain to delivering a timely response. These include: (i) inadequate resources to deliver interventions at large scale; (ii) inadequate staffing levels and training in public health analysis and decisionmaking at all levels; and (iii) inadequate salaries at all levels to allow public health officials to adequately perform their public health functions rather than focusing on income generation.

Surveillance systems for drug use, HIV/AIDS and STIs continue to depend on compulsory notification/registration systems and outdated screening programs which persist from the Soviet era. CDC is developing sites for quality controlled laboratories in Osh and Bishkek (primarily testing for HIV and hepatitis markers) and linking these to prevalence and behavioral surveys among risk groups. There is an urgent need to ensure that sentinel and second-generation surveillance approaches continue to be supported and extended as new waves of harm reduction and prevention projects reach new geographic locations and risk sub-groups. There is currently no sentinel surveillance for STIs. Better use could be made of existing data screening population segments to gain insights into HIV and STI prevalence rates.

Kyrgyz Republic: Key Indicators at a Glance (2003–2004)	
AIDS/HIV Deaths*	22
AIDS Cases—Cumulative*	31
AIDS Cases—New*	10
HIV Cases—Cumulative*	655
HIV Cases—Cumulative/100,000	11.5
Increase HIV—Cum 2000–2003	9.3 fold
M:F Ratio HIV—Cumulative	
Proportion of HIV Cumulative among 20–29yr old	
HIV Cumulative among IDU	410
HIV Cases—New*	161
Proportion of New HIV acquired through IDU*	77.1%
HIV Cases—New/100,000	3.1
M:F Ratio New Cases	5.9
Highest Oblast new HIV rate	Osh
New HIV /100,000 (all ages) in Highest Oblast	6.29
Estimated HIV Prevalence IDU	1.3
Estimated HIV Prevalence Prisoners (males)	0.74
Estimated prevalence in pregnant women*	11
Registered Drug Users	6,327
M:F Sex Ratio Drug Users	14:1
Registered IDU	
Estimated IDU	70,000
Estimated HIV Preval. IDU	4,400
Estimated CSW	5,000′
Estimated MSM	30,000′

*Figures for 2004.

HIV/AIDS and STIs in the Kyrgyz Republic: Epidemiological Trends

Drug Use. There has been a five-fold increase in registered drugs users (RDU) since the beginning of the 1990s although the rate of increase has declined between 2002 and 2003. Estimates of a total number of drug users of around 100,000 (1.25 per 100,000) are consistent with all available data. Around 70 percent of these are IDUs. Men still predominate with a sex ratio among registered drug users above 14:1. The proportion of drug users injecting and using heroin has increased. Among males in their 30s, the registration rate per 100,000 approaches 1 percent of the total population of that age. When age and sex distributions for the whole country are applied to the cases occurring in Bishkek and Osh, among men in their 30s the registration rates are respectively in excess of 1.5 percent and 2 percent of the population. Numbers and rates of currently registered drug users for the last 13 years are shown in Figure 6. It shows a 4.5-fold increase in RDUs since the beginning of the 1990s. Since 2001, after a sharp decrease during 1998–2000, the number of RDUs has continued to increase at a rate of about 600 per year reaching a total number of 6,327 people in 2003, or around 126 per 100,000. Of these, 4,400 (70 percent) were injecting drug users; 4,009

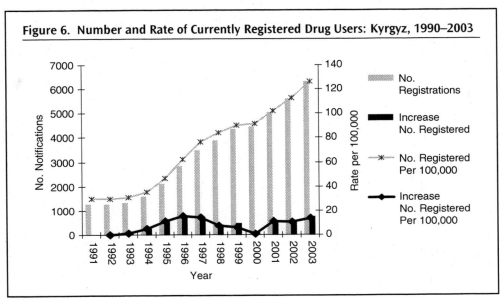

Figure 6. Number and Rate of Currently Registered Drug Users: Kyrgyz, 1990–2003

Source: MoH Kyrgyz Republic.

(63 percent) were opiate users; and 1,702 (27 percent) were heroin users. The male:female ratio was 14:1. UNODC has estimated that around 6 percent of drug users in the country are registered. If this is the case, then the total number of drug users is around 105,000, which is 2,100 drug users per 100,000 population, or 2 percent of the total population.

Figures 7 shows the number of RDUs by region. Figure 8 shows the geographical distribution of RDUs per 100,000 population between 1991 and 2003. The highest

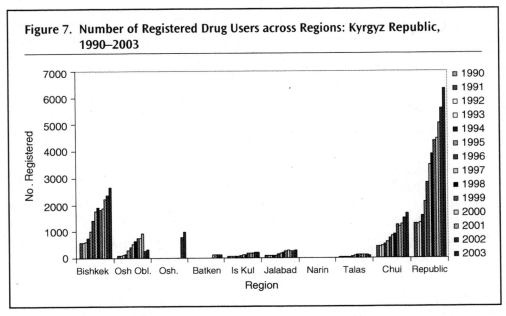

Figure 7. Number of Registered Drug Users across Regions: Kyrgyz Republic, 1990–2003

Source: MoH Kyrgyz Republic.

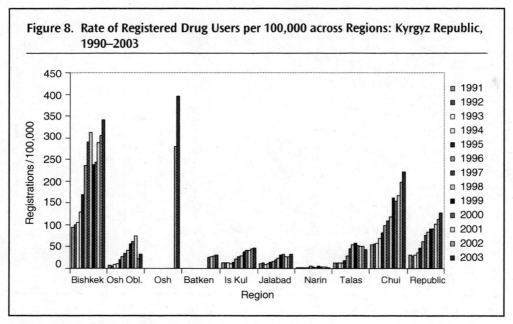

Figure 8. Rate of Registered Drug Users per 100,000 across Regions: Kyrgyz Republic, 1990–2003

Source: MoH Kyrgyz Republic.

number of registrations throughout the period was in Bishkek. However, the rate of RDUs appears to be higher in Osh, although the data exist only for the last two years. In Osh in 2003 the rate of RDUs reached 394/100,000. Chui oblast shows consistently high rates of RDUs.

Examination of the age distribution of registrations and registration rates of drug use in the country (Figure 9) also highlights some remarkable results. Among males in their 30s, the registration rate per 100,000 approaches 1 percent of the total population of that age. When age and sex distributions for the whole country are applied to the cases occurring in Bishkek and Osh, among men in their 30s the registration rates are respectively in excess of 1.5 percent and 2 percent of the population (Figure 10).

HIV/AIDS. Although a total of 15 HIV cases were identified and registered in the Republic between 1987 and 1991, the Republican AIDS Center (RAC) reports that these all occurred among individuals of Asian and African origin who were not Kyrgyz or from the USSR. The RAC also reports that of the remaining 36 cases of HIV infection identified and registered at the end of 2000, 23 were from CIS countries (16 from Russia, 4 from Ukraine, 2 from Kazakhstan, and 1 from Uzbekistan). No cases of HIV infection were identified between 1991 and 1994. Current Government estimates put the number of persons living with HIV in the Kyrgyz Republic at almost 500, with over 85 percent of HIV-positive persons believed to be drug users. Cumulative cases increased rapidly since 1996 to reach 494 (11.5 per 100,000) by the end of 2003. The number of new cases has stabilized around 150 cases per year (3 per 100,000) over the last 3 years. In 2002, 113 drug users were tested positive for HIV infection, representing 85 percent of new cases.

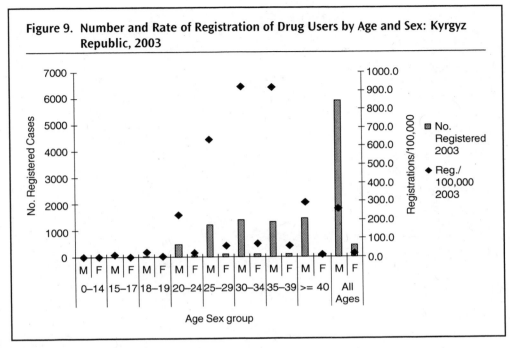

Figure 9. Number and Rate of Registration of Drug Users by Age and Sex: Kyrgyz Republic, 2003

Source: MoH Kyrgyz Republic.

The male:female ratio among new cases in 2002 was 5:9. There have been no recorded cases of transmission through homosexual sex. There is a wide variation in HIV notification rates by region. Prevalence among IDUs across the country is probably still below 2 percent. In Osh City, the prevalence of HIV infection in males may exceed 0.1 percent overall and 0.5 percent among men aged 20–29. The prevalence in prisons is probably still below 1 percent.

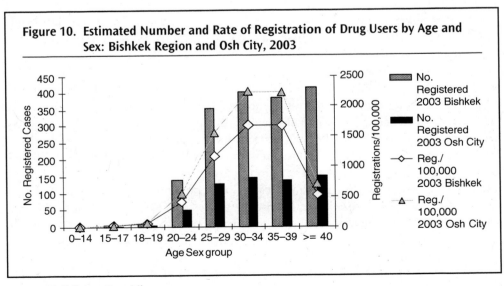

Figure 10. Estimated Number and Rate of Registration of Drug Users by Age and Sex: Bishkek Region and Osh City, 2003

Source: MoH Kyrgyz Republic.

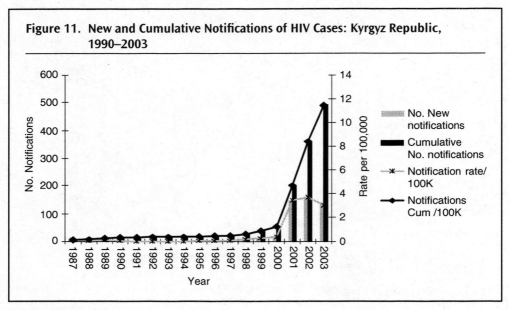

Figure 11. New and Cumulative Notifications of HIV Cases: Kyrgyz Republic, 1990–2003

Source: MoH Kyrgyz Republic.

Figure 12 shows the regional distribution of the number and rate of notifications in the Kyrgyz Republic between 2001 and 2003. UNAIDS has estimated that the true number of cases of HIV infection may be 10 times the number of notified cases (Kyrgyz Republic CCM 2002). The figure shows that Osh Oblast (mainly the city) had the highest rate of infection in the country in the last three years: it was 2 to 3 times higher than the rate registered in the capital. The official data use as denominator the population of the entire Oblast. If population of the Osh city alone is used as denominator, the rate for 2001 would approach 50 per 100,000. In the Bishkek Narcology Dispensary, in 2003 out of 147 patients tested for HIV 2 were positive.

STI. Syphilis incidence increased from 12 per 100,000 in 1990, to 368 per 100,000 in 1996, but then decreased to stabilize around 42 per 100,000 in 2002–2003. Thus, the size of the epidemic has been large and distributed widely throughout the whole country. It is not clear to what extent the decline in syphilis notifications since the mid 1990s reflects a true decrease in incidence and/or declining visits to medical facilities and consequently, declining notification. Prevalence of syphilis among CSWs may be above 30 percent and among prisoners above 3 percent. The number of notifications of new cases of syphilis for each year between 1990 and 2003 for each region is presented in Figure 13. The Figure shows a very rapid increase in incidence throughout the early 1990s with a peak in 1996–97 in all regions. The largest number of cases occurred in Bishkek, Osh and Chui regions. The corresponding notification rates per 100,000 populations are shown in Figure 14.

The data suggest an epidemic fairly evenly distributed across the country, although there is a clear concentration in the capital, Bishkek. In 1993, the overall notification rate exceeded 350 per 100,000 total population in Bishkek. This translates into a rate of about

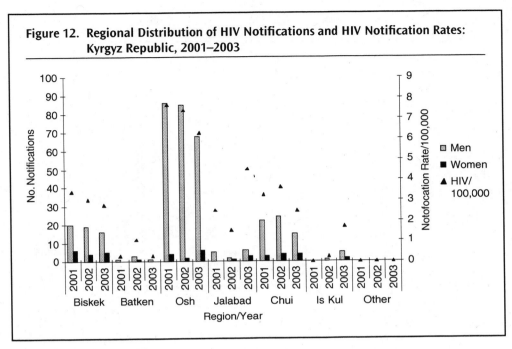

Figure 12. Regional Distribution of HIV Notifications and HIV Notification Rates: Kyrgyz Republic, 2001–2003

Source: MoH Kyrgyz Republic.

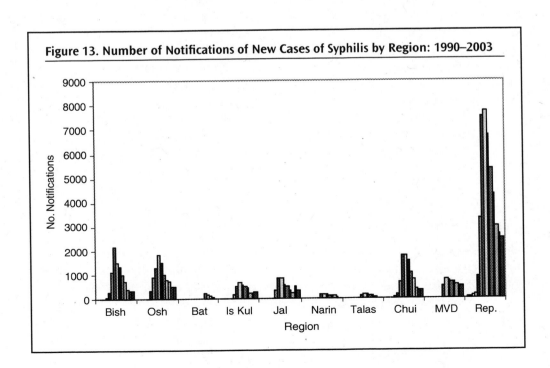

Figure 13. Number of Notifications of New Cases of Syphilis by Region: 1990–2003

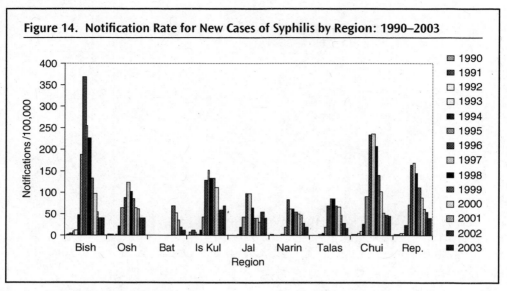

Figure 14. Notification Rate for New Cases of Syphilis by Region: 1990–2003

Source: MoH of the Kyrgyz Republic.

1 percent in the sexually active population; and it is likely that rates among 15–30 year olds exceeded 2 percent this year. It seems likely that the decline after the mid 1990s represents a combination of a real decline in the incidence of syphilis, together with a decrease in the proportion of case notifications due to changing patterns of clinical care. Data describing age distribution suggest that around 5 percent of cases are persons who are less than 17 years old; 6 percent are among 18–19 year-olds; 46 percent are among 20–29 year-olds; 30 percent are among 30–39 year-olds and 13 percent are 40 and above. Published evidence suggests that in 1999 the notification rate among pregnant women was 345 per 100,000 and that almost half of syphilis cases in that year occurred among the homeless or unemployed.

A survey carried out among CSWs in 1998 suggested a prevalence of syphilis of 16 percent. In addition, data on STI prevalence among CSWs at a special clinic run for these women in Bishkek are available. Among first time visitors in 2001, 38 percent had syphilis; 5 percent gonorrhea; 12 percent trichomonas; and 14 percent chlamydia.

Risk Behavior and Environment

The Kyrgyz Republic is a small, poor, mountainous country with a predominantly agricultural economy. Cotton, wool, and meat are the main agricultural products and exports. Industrial exports include gold, mercury, uranium, and electricity. The Kyrgyz Republic has been one of the most progressive countries of the former Soviet Union in carrying out market reforms. Following a successful stabilization program, which lowered inflation from 88 percent to 15 percent in 1997, attention is turning toward stimulating growth. Most of the Government's stocks in enterprises have been sold. Drops in production had been severe since the break-up of the Soviet Union in December 1991, but by mid-1995 production began to recover and exports began to increase. With a declining GDP per capita (from $503 in 1992 to $308 in 2001) has come a decline in funds available for the health sector (World Bank 2004a).

Although there has been strong support for the economy through international aid and financial assistance, many elements of the old Soviet health and social infrastructure have experienced considerable decline. However, the Kyrgyz Government's response has been much more reform oriented than that of its neighbors and this has included significant achievements in health sector reforms and the development of primary care. Kyrgyzstan's openness to reform has put its leaders across sectors in touch with modern thinking in relation to public health theory and practice, and this has been reflected in an innovative and proactive approach to the control of STIs and HIV/AIDS. However, there are still significant challenges posed by lack of sufficient levels of resources and continued need for reforms in the economy as well as health and other social sectors.

Like its neighbors, Kyrgyzstan has experienced an explosion in injecting drug use and commercial sex work with the development of local markets for transited opiates from Afghanistan, since the early 1990s; and consequently, HIV/AIDS outbreaks have been reported in the main cities across the country. There are strong indications that the size of highly-vulnerable groups for HIV—IDUs, CSWs, MSM, migrants, and prisoners—has seen a rapid increase over the recent years. There are approximately 80,000–100,000 IDUs and 3,000 CSWs in the country and levels of risk behavior appear to be high (Kyrgyz CCM 2002).

Anecdotal data and rapid assessment suggest that there have been very large increases in the number of IDUs, CSWs, and migrants over the last 10 years in the country (UNAIDS 2002c). Increased income differentials and poverty create demand for and supply of CSWs; while the passage of drug trafficking routes carrying opiates through the country delivers a copious supply of cheap opium and heroin to fuel the epidemics of injecting drug use. Hostile and dishonest police behavior in relation to CSWs and IDUs is present through-out the country, driving them into patterns of behavior associated with very high risks of HIV transmission. High levels of migration, including to destinations with higher background prevalence of HIV infection, are likely to continue seeding infection into the general population. A decline in social support services and participation in education as well as widespread unemployment leave young people increasingly vulnerable to risk behavior associated with HIV infection.

The Government has been a leader in the region in taking early actions directed toward the mitigation of these threats. Considerable work has been done towards delivering and creating a facilitative environment for harm reduction and other interventions among highly vulnerable groups. Having repealed the law criminalizing homosexuality in 1997 and the law on voluntary adult prostitution in 1998, the parliament allowed the start of coherent HIV/AIDS prevention programs among MSM and CSWs (Basmavoka and others 2003). However, a legal basis for the compulsory testing of "risk groups" including IDUs, CSWs, and prisoners still remains, and the provision and uptake of VCT are still very low. There remains, therefore, a need both for further revisions in legislation and an expansion of efforts to change the attitudes and behavior of police towards highly vulnerable groups.

Several surveys have attempted to characterize the public attitudes and knowledge concerning HIV, STIs, and risk groups. They have consistently found high levels of negative attitudes to risk groups, including MSM, CSWs, and IDUs. Levels of knowledge about HIV risks and transmission routes are still low: only 68 percent of respondents are able to identify condoms as a means for protection against HIV and other STIs, and only 40 percent know that HIV could be transmitted through injecting drugs (Basmakova and others 2003).

The number of registered drug users continues to increase, and evidence points to over 100,000 drug users, of which perhaps 70,000 are injecting drug users and 65,000 opiate users. According to some evidence, previously high levels of risk behavior, including sharing of syringes, may be decreasing. Rates of injecting drug use are far higher among men than among women, but it is likely that figures for women are estimated less accurately in routine data-gathering process. Drug users are becoming younger, and there are reports of a shift away from traditional opium injection to heroin injection. The current extent to which injecting drug users engage in commercial sex work to earn money to purchase drugs is unknown; but early research suggested it was a common practice among female IDUs in Osh (Express 1998).

In 2000, an attempt was made to carry out a prevalence survey by examining residues in syringes obtained through needle exchange returns. Initial estimates of prevalence of HIV among IDUs of 14 percent in Bishkek and 40 percent in Osh have proved suspect; validation tests suggest that the results are not interpretable. Behavioral information was also collected and it is described below. An interview was conducted with 68 men and 32 women. The following are their demographic and social characteristics: 83 percent of the interviewed were less than 35 years old; 57 percent were unemployed; 74 percent were single; 61 percent were Russian, 9 percent Kyrgyz, and 30 percent of other nationalities. According to the results of the interviews, 53 percent of men and women in this group had their first experience with drugs before they had turned 18. Distribution of duration of injecting drug use was the following: 48 percent of those interviewed had been injecting drugs for 5 years or less; 48 percent from 5 to 20 years; and 4 percent for 20 to 30 years. Of these, 92 percent used opiates, (70–80 percent opium). Only 20 percent used sterile syringes; 29 percent used the same syringe on multiple occasions; and 51 percent used any syringes; 67 percent used boiled water to sterilize equipment; 72 percent injected 2 to 5 times a day; 46 percent used drugs in groups; 64 percent thought syringes were too expensive; 91 percent were sexually active; and 55 percent reported that their sexual partners used condoms; 46 percent, however, never used condoms; while 12 percent used condoms all the time; 55 percent of the sample used sex as an income source (both men and women); 85 percent of respondents gave a positive evaluation of syringe exchange points; 5 percent said they did not need them; while 48 percent wanted them to be closer to their homes; 25 percent wanted syringes delivered to their homes; and 18 percent wanted syringes to be given in pharmacies for free.

A followup survey was conducted in December 2000. The most considerable change was observed in the kind of addictions. The majority of IDUs (70–80 percent) used opium during the period that the survey took place. In December, 73 percent of those polled used heroin as opposed to 26 percent who used opium. This is an unfavorable tendency among the Bishkek IDU population. Those who turned to needle exchange services showed a considerable reduction in risk behavior in relation to injecting drug use. Significant increases in condom use were also observed. In 2001, two samples of 100 injecting drug users were recruited from needle exchange points in Bishkek and Chui oblast (area 1): one at the beginning and one at the end of the year. One person only was found to be HIV positive.

Behavioral information was also collected from this group. Methods used for injections became significantly safer: 68 percent reported using only sterile syringes; 13 percent said they sometimes shared syringes; 71 percent used syringes no more than twice and 26 percent 3–5 times; 66 percent wanted to get off drugs, while 25 percent did not (mainly younger and more recent addicts). Thirteen men died in the first 3 months of 2001, compared with 7 in 2000 from overdose.

The number of CSWs in the country is unknown. However estimates suggest that there may be some 1,600–3,000 in Bishkek City; 750 in Osh City; and 200 in Jalalabad (Oostvogels 1999; Basmakova and others 2003). This would suggest that there may be up to 5,000 CSWs countrywide. The daily turnover of their clientele is approximately one to two clients per one CSW. Available reports also estimate fast growth of the CSW population, with a turnover rate of 40 percent a year. There is a high rate of unsafe sexual behavior among CSWs, which potentially could contribute to the spread of HIV epidemic. It is likely that a significant number of CSWs in the country may be using drugs in various ways. The Government's application to the GFATM indicates that over half of CSW do not use condoms, and that 10 to 30 percent may provide sex in exchange for drugs (Kyrgyz Republic CCM 2002). An assessment of CSWs in Bishkek revealed that 49 percent were migrants who came to the city in search of a better life (Kyrgyz Republic and UNDP 2003).

It has been estimated that there are at least 100 men selling sex to men in Biskek (Basmakova and others 2003). The Government estimates that there may be 30,000 MSM in the country. Otherwise, there is very little information concerning the numbers of MSM in the Kyrgyz Republic or their behavior. Homosexuality remains highly stigmatized. Bishkek is best studied in this respect and targeted AIDS prevention programs are carried out covering 5,000 MSM. Joint expert assessment performed in Osh by international and national experts showed significant numbers of MSM in Osh region as well as high levels of unsafe sexual behavior among them.

Among the 419 Kyrgyz citizens registered as HIV positive by the end of 2003, 56 percent were identified among the prison population. According to official reports, prisons are a major source for HIV/AIDS. The prevalence of HIV among prisoners is estimated at 776.4 per 100,000, which is 131.6 times higher than among the adult population in the country. The very high incidence rate of TB in prisons (about 2,000 per 100,000) with increasing prevalence of HIV, further increases the health risks among the prison population. The reported prevalence of syphilis among prisoners was also reported to be very high at approximately 3,500 per 100,000 population (3.5 percent), which is 70 times higher than among the general population of the country (Godinho and others 2004). According to an anonymous survey among the prison inmates and the wardens conducted in 2002, drugs are accessible in all correction facilities, and 70 to 80 percent of prisoners inject drugs. Therefore, there is a real danger of rapid spread of HIV, hepatitis, syphilis and other infections in prisons in the Kyrgyz Republic (Kyrgyz Republic CCM 2002).

The Kyrgyz Republic has been experiencing considerable external and internal migration, especially from rural areas to big cities. The migrant population seems to be an important target group for HIV control. External migration in the country amounts to 50,000 people a year (including immigrants and emigrants), who mainly leave or come from CIS countries (Kyrgyz Republic and UNDP 2003). The number of internal migrants is also significant. Due to their precarious circumstances, migrants are vulnerable to high-risk behavior such as commercial sex and IDU.

Prevention and Control

Surveillance. Surveillance of drug use and dependency is carried out through the usual system of registration of clinically confirmed cases by clinicians working in Narcology Services. There is a statutory obligation for physicians to maintain on this register newly identified individuals until they meet formal criteria for removal. Registration rates clearly underestimate the prevalence of drug use in the country, but UNODC (2003) estimates that 6 percent of all drug users may be registered in treatment.

Routine HIV surveillance is carried out through health service structures in testing laboratories located mostly in the AIDS centers. The samples originate from clinical and population groups and blood donations. Tested groups include: registered drug users, patients with STI diagnoses, and pregnant women. Testing is irregular—it varies in particular with test availability. The number of routine tests performed has declined since the early 1990s stabilizing at about 140,000 tests per year in 1997. A total of 137,781 tests were carried out in 2003, less than half of which were of blood donations. On average, more than 15,000 persons with clinical indications, an STI, or pregnancy are tested each year. The numbers of patients tested anonymously has increased over recent years. Positive ELISA tests are required to be confirmed by Western Blot. Identified HIV infected persons are invited to attend clinical services where an epidemiological interview is conducted to establish key demographic variables and likely route of transmission. Completed information on HIV positive individuals put in standard notification forms and statistical summaries is then sent to the center. The extent to which numbers and trends in notified cases reflect the true incidence or prevalence of HIV/AIDS in the country is limited by both variation in numbers and 'case mix' of individuals tested each year.

The Kyrgyz Republic, as other countries in the region, continues to use a system of notification by a clinician of clinically confirmed cases of sexually transmitted infection as the primary means of STI surveillance. During the Soviet period this system probably identified the majority of diagnosed cases of syphilis. However, since 1990 it is highly likely that there has been a decline in the accuracy of notification rates as a result of an increasing tendency among patients to use paid anonymous services obtained in the public or private sector. The problem is worsened as a result of a squeeze on funding for the STI structures, a lack of availability of sensitive and specific diagnostic tests, and strict case definitions for reporting which do not reflect the fact that cases may be syndromically diagnosed and managed. In addition there has been a planned cutback in the size of the Dermatological and Venereal Disease Service, with some shifting of STI diagnosis and management into primary care, supported by the development and introduction of protocols for syndromic management in areas where diagnostic tests are simply unavailable. Reliable syphilis diagnostic services are available in urban centers but there are no reliable tests available for chlamydia or gonorrhea infections in women.

With the support of CDC and USAID, the country is moving towards adoption of sentinel surveillance within the framework of Second-Generation HIV Surveillance recommended by WHO/UNAIDS (2000). Sites that are currently under development are Bishkek and Osh, though the stage of development is behind that which has been obtained in Kazakhstan. The focus will be on supporting development of laboratory capacity for HIV and hepatitis testing (with some work also on syphilis diagnostics) and quality control systems. Trainings as well as systematic evaluation of the sensitivity and specificity of diagnostics produced in the region will be delivered. In addition, prevalence surveys linked to behavioral surveys will be carried out among risk groups in collaboration with outreach and harm-reduction projects.

Prevention among Vulnerable Groups. Harm reduction projects comprising needle exchange, outreach, health education, and condom provision have operated in the country since the late 1990s. There are three needle exchange points operating in Bishkek, one in Tokmok, and two in Osh. In addition, three more are programmed for Bishkek and one more for Jalalabad. Support for these has been provided primarily from OSI. These projects have done significant amount of work to change police attitudes to IDUs, including running of training seminars and roundtables, and publishing a manual for police officers. Support groups for police have been set up and training of judges and prosecutors will commence in 2004. In 2003, one needle exchange site in Bishkek served 1,090 persons; 30 percent of which were women. CSWs comprised approximately one third of all women who attended this site. Less than half (40 percent) of the IDUs who used these needle exchange services were registered at the Narcology Services. There are also several condom distribution and sexual health promotion activities. Some harm reduction projects are starting to employ dermato-venereal disease specialists to provide on-site sexual health and STI advice.

Innovative work with CSWs is also moving forward. In 2004, the Tais plus NGO with support from WHO launched a program linked to outreach activities in Bishkek that provides IEC, condom promotion, clinical STI diagnosis and treatment services, and peer education to CSWs. A pilot MSM prevention project was developed in Bishkek through the NGO Oasis in 1998–1999 with WHO support. The project has carried out outreach, IEC and condom promotion activities and provided a help line and educational and cultural events for MSM. Informal MSM groups have been identified or established. It is estimated that 350 MSM have been contacted and there were 1,233 contacts to the hotline (Basmakova and others 2003). Fifty seven thousand condoms were distributed by the project to MSM in 2001–2002. However, UNICEF's attempt to update the sexual health education in schools in 2003 backfired, and the Ministry of Health did not allow the adoption of a new textbook including education on safe sex and HIV/AIDS.

Clinical and Laboratory Services. There are two Narcology Dispensaries with 285 beds and a total of 102 narcologists (50 percent full time). There is also a network of consultation centers throughout the country. The main clinical services provided are detoxification with little social or psychological support. Patients pay on average 1,010 Soms (about $24) for 21 days of in-patient detoxification course. Current legislation requires registration of all patients, which results in their exclusion from certain types of employment. Anonymous services can be obtained, but they are expensive. The service estimates that 30 percent of female IDUs are also CSWs, and that the current needle exchange program meets only 6 to 10 percent of total need. Recently, the Narcology Service has been involved in management and delivery of needle exchange services and in supporting self-help groups (Narcotics Anonymous). Residential rehabilitation is available but it is expensive being provided only in the private sector. Narcologists have been involved in the development of the GFATM-financed program and considerable resources were earmarked within the grant for diversification of drug services. Two pilot methadone substitution therapy programs have started working in the Kyrgyz Republic since 2002: one in Osh and one in Bishkek. Their introduction was preceded by lengthy disputes between the Drug Control Agency, the Ministry of Health, doctors, NGOs, and the Police, but they are under implementation now.

Clinical and laboratory services for HIV/AIDS are provided through the National AIDS Centre, five regional AIDS Centers (in Issyk-Kul, Naryn, Talas, Osh, and Jalalabad), and 36 HIV diagnostic laboratories. Three more AIDS Centers (in Chui, Batken, and Bishkek City) are being opened. These centers provide HIV testing (including screening predetermined risk groups as well as blood donations), some counseling, and treatment for HIV-related disease. They also conduct epidemiological interviews with individuals who test HIV positive. The AIDS structures have committed themselves to expanding VCT services. There is a network of individuals trained in psychosocial counseling on HIV/AIDS. Facilities where anonymous HIV tests can be obtained are also becoming available. However, coverage is poor and the number individuals tested through VCT has been very small. Throughout the country there are continuing problems with supplies of basic medical and laboratory equipment and donor blood is inconsistently screened. Only palliative treatment is available for HIV infected individuals and there is very little use of antiretroviral drugs (ARVs; Basmakova and others 2003).

Until 2000, the STI services continued to be based broadly on the old Soviet model, with each of the six oblasts having its own Oblast Dispensary and associated services. However, with the shift towards the development of primary care the system has been restructured. There are now two dispensaries, the Republican Dispensary in Bishkek and the Oblast Dispensary in Osh (1992: 10), with 169 dermato-venereologists (1992: 264) and 597 beds (1992: 1,185). Dermatological and Venereal Disease Units are now established in general hospitals and polyclinics. In addition, there has been some attempt to introduce syndromic diagnosis of STIs given frequent shortages of diagnostic tests. On the one hand, improved availability and acceptability of services might have increased diagnosis, but on the other hand, absence of a microscopic, serological or microbiological diagnosis has been undermining these achievements.

Active case-finding through screening occupational and clinical groups is declining. However, 80 percent of syphilis is currently detected through contact-tracing from index cases; and 20 percent through self-referral. There has been a variety of pilots of syndromic diagnosis and management including the MSF supported project in Osh. The Republican DV Dispensary provides clinical services to the CSW project in Bishkek. Essential STI drugs are widely available in Bishkek, but there are reports of shortages in the periphery. Patients pay for all treatments. Given the unusual flexibility and openness to modernization demonstrated by the Dermatological and Venereal Disease service, and the shift in focus of provision to primary care structures, there is scope for funding further development of innovative services for risk groups through this service. At the country level, ensuring that information about STIs and ways to access confidential STI services are incorporated as key elements into harm reduction and outreach projects among CSWs, drug users and migrants should be one of the priorities.

Key Findings in Tajikistan

The total number of registered drug users more than doubled from 2,905 in 1999 (45 per 100,000) to 6,356 (99 per 100,000) in 2001. The share of RDUs using heroin rose from 63 percent to 75 percent over the same period. Around 70 percent of these are IDUs. The estimated registration rate for opiate users among 18–35 year-old men in Dushanbe is of 3.5 percent. Current Government estimates put the number of persons living with HIV in Tajikistan at 119 (1.9 per 100,000), with over 75 percent of HIV-positive persons believed to be drug users. New cases identified have risen steadily over the same period with 42 cases

Tajikistan: Key Indicators at a Glance (2003)	
AIDS/HIV Deaths	0
AIDS Cases—Cumulative	1
AIDS Cases—New	1
HIV Cases—Cumulative	119
HIV Cases—Cumulative/100,000	1.8
Increase HIV—Cum. 2000–2003	17 fold
M:F Ratio HIV—Cumulative	
Proportion of HIV Cumulative among 20–29 yr. olds	51%
HIV Cumulative among IDU	88
HIV Cases—New	42
Proportion of New HIV acquired through IDU	75%
HIV Cases—New/100,000	0.7
M:F Ratio New Cases	7.4
Highest Oblast new HIV rate	
New HIV/100,000 (all ages) in Highest Oblast	
Estimated HIV Prevalence IDU	0.5%
Estimated HIV Prevalence Prisoners (males)	0.74
Estimated prevalence in pregnant women	
Registered Drug Users	6,356
M:F Sex Ratio Drug Users	18:1
Registered IDU	
Estimated IDU	58,000
Estimated HIV Preval. IDU	0.5
Estimated CSW	5,000'
Estimated MSM	

(0.7 per 100,000) identified in 2003. In 2003, only 1 out of 400 drug users tested for HIV in the Narcology Services was found positive for HIV. Prevalence among IDUs across the country is probably still below 2 percent. Notified syphilis cases increased from 107 (1.6 per 100,000) in 1990 to 1320 (23.8 per 100,000) in 1998 falling to 778 (12.3 per 100,000) in 2003; with significant epidemic occurring in all regions. It is not clear to what extent the decline in syphilis notification since the mid-1990s reflects a true decrease in incidence and/or declining visits to official facilities and notification.

The Government of Tajikistan has tried to respond to the increase in HIV infection rates and to mitigate consequences of drug use. It has approved a Strategic Plan, obtained a GFATM grant in the first round, and has recently submitted a new grant proposal as the first grant has been almost entirely disbursed. However, implementation of the National Program on HIV/AIDS and STIs has been slow. Relative to the threat that Tajikistan faces, current interventions to avert the generalized epidemic and their coverage are largely inadequate. An encouraging sign has been the recent expansion of the NGO sector. There are currently more than a thousand NGOs registered in Tajikistan, although it is not clear how many of these are operational or funded. However, NGOs are certainly active among populations vulnerable to heroin use.

Surveillance for HIV, STIs and drug use continue to depend on compulsory notification/registration systems and outdated screening programs which persist from the Soviet era. Surveillance of drug use and dependency is carried out through the usual system of registration of clinically confirmed cases by clinicians working in Narcology Services. There is a statutory obligation for physicians to maintain in this register newly identified individuals until they meet formal criteria for removal. Registration rates clearly underestimate the prevalence of drug use in the country. According to UNODC estimates (2003), 8 percent of all drug users are registered for treatment.

HIV/AIDS and STIs in Tajikistan: Epidemiological Trends

Drug Use. Total numbers of registered drug users more than doubled from 2,905 in 1999 (45 per 100,000) to 6,356 (99 per 100,000) in 2001. Around 90 percent of RDUs used opiates throughout the period, but the proportion using heroin rose from 63 percent to 75 percent. The male/female ratio declined from 35 to 17 over the same period. Around 70 percent of these are IDUs. The highest number of cases were reported in Dushanbe, where the number of registered male opiate users exceeded 3,126 (1,112 per 100,000) in 2001, which is over 1 percent of the total male population. These very high rates of drug use become even more astonishing when we stratify notification rates by age and region. The registration rate for opiate users among 18 to 35 year-old men in Dushanbe is 3.5 percent. The number of registered drug users and rates per 100,000 are shown in Figure 15.

The age distribution of registered cases and rate is shown in Figure 16. The majority of RDUs in all years are 18 to 30 years old. The geographical distribution of registered opiate users in 2000 and 2001 is shown in Figure 17.

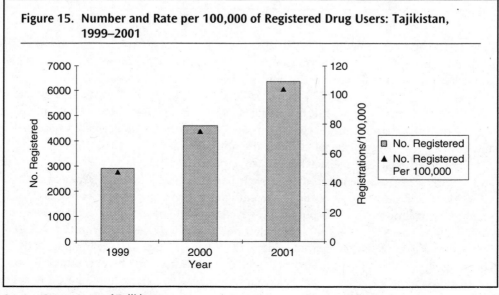

Figure 15. Number and Rate per 100,000 of Registered Drug Users: Tajikistan, 1999–2001

Source: Government of Tajikistan.

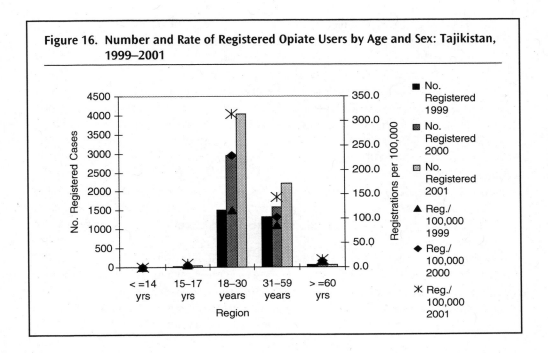

Figure 16. Number and Rate of Registered Opiate Users by Age and Sex: Tajikistan, 1999–2001

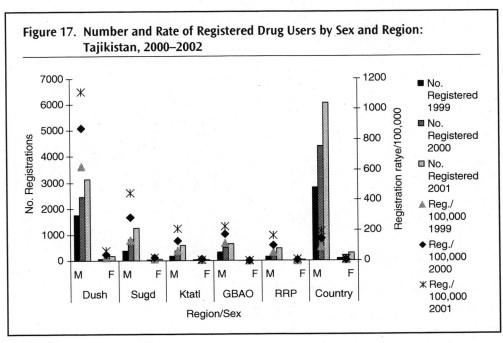

Figure 17. Number and Rate of Registered Drug Users by Sex and Region: Tajikistan, 2000–2002

Source: Government of Tajikistan.

HIV/AIDS. According to Government estimates in 2003, the number of people living with HIV in Tajikistan was 119 (1.9 per 100,000). Identification of new cases rose steadily over the same period with 42 cases (0.7 per 100,000) identified in 2003. In 2002, in 75 percent of notified cases the infection was acquired through IDU and in 14 percent of cases through sexual transmission. The male:female ratio for cumulative cases at the end of 2003 was 3.6:1 and for new cases identified in 2003 it was 7.4:1. There is a wide variation in HIV notification rates by region, with the highest rate observed in Dushanbe. In 2003, one out of 400 drug users tested positive for HIV at the Narcology Services. Prevalence among IDUs across the country is probably still below 2 percent. Availability of HIV tests has been highly restricted. In 2003, 42 new cases were identified increasing the total number of cases in the country to 119 cases. The true number of cases is likely to be significantly higher. Due to increased availability and use of testing, in January 2004 alone, 33 new cases were identified, suggesting existence of a significant hidden epidemic in the country. A majority of those tested positive are IDUs.

The number of new notifications and rates per 100,000 total population, together with cumulative HIV notifications and notification rates are shown in Figure 18. Cumulative cases have increased rapidly since 1999. According to Government experts, taking into account that medical examination among vulnerable groups is not conducted the real number of HIV infected individuals is ten, and in some regions 20 times higher (Tajik CCM 2004).

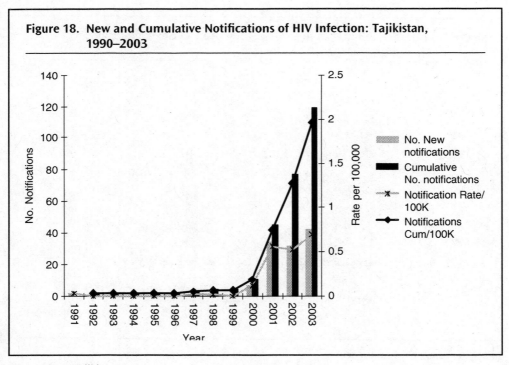

Figure 18. New and Cumulative Notifications of HIV Infection: Tajikistan, 1990–2003

Source: MoH Tajikistan.

Table 12. Age and Sex Distribution of Cases of HIV Infection Notified: Tajikistan 1991–2003

Age	1991		1997		1998		2000		2001		2002		2003		Total
	M	F	M	F	M	F	M	F	M	F	M	F	M	F	
0–4											1				1
5–14											2				2
15–19							2		2	2					6
20–29			1		1		2		12	8	9	4	17	5	59
30–39							2		5	2	12	2	16		39
40–49	2							1	1	1	1	1	3		10
50–59									1				1		2
>=60															0
Subtotal	2	0	1	0	1	0	6	1	21	13	25	7	37	5	119
Total	2		1		1		7		34		32		42		119

Source: MoH Tajikistan.

Table 12 shows the age and sex distribution of HIV infection notifications in Tajikistan for the past twelve years.

STIs. Notified syphilis cases increased from 107 (1.6 per 100,000) in 1990 to 1,320 (23.8 per 100,000) in 1998 falling to 778 (12.3 per 100,000) in 2003, with significant epidemic occurring in all regions. Figure 18 shows the number of new cases of syphilis registered in Tajikistan between 1990 and 2003. The figure shows a clear concentration of the epidemic in the capital, Dushanbe, where the notification rate reached almost 90 per 100,000 in 1995. There were six cases of congenital syphilis in 2003. These suggest significant epidemics of the full range of STIs. The size of the syphilis epidemic in Tajikistan has been much smaller than in other countries in the region (about half the size of that experienced in Turkmenistan and Uzbekistan and about one-tenth the size of those in Kazakhstan and the Kyrgyz Republic). It is not clear whether this smaller size and the decline since 1997 reflect a real decline in incidence or changes in service accessibility and/or accuracy in notification.

Risk Behavior and Environment

Tajikistan is among the poorest countries in the world. It was also the poorest republic in the former Soviet Union, and still has the lowest GDP of the 15 former Soviet republics. Since 1991, it has experienced three changes in government and a five-year civil war (1992–1997) responsible for over 60,000 deaths, countless rapes, and the displacement of as many as one million people. The war caused thousands of ethnic minorities, including key professionals in industry, construction, transportation and engineering, to permanently emigrate. Peace accords were signed in 1997 and a power-sharing mechanism

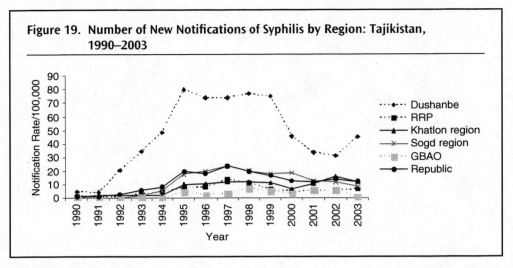

Figure 19. Number of New Notifications of Syphilis by Region: Tajikistan, 1990–2003

Source: Government of Tajikistan.

known as the National Reconciliation Commission was established. The civil war destroyed the already weak economy—particularly in southern and eastern regions—generated paramilitary gangs who now struggle for control of the illicit drug trade.

Tajikistan's population is young and mostly rural: 43 percent of its population is 15 years or younger; and 73 percent resides in rural areas. The poverty level is high with 80 percent of the population living below the poverty line. Inflation in 2001 was 33 percent and real unemployment is high. It is estimated that between 30 and 50 percent of the country's economy is linked to drug trafficking. The transition to a market economy has reduced the number of

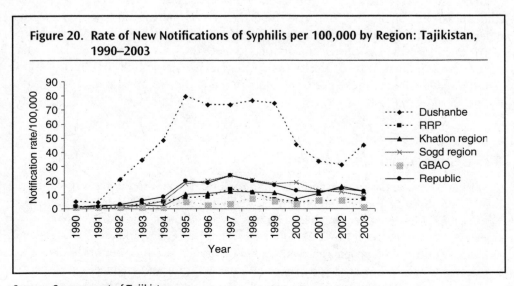

Figure 20. Rate of New Notifications of Syphilis per 100,000 by Region: Tajikistan, 1990–2003

Source: Government of Tajikistan.

government jobs by half. GDP per capita fell from $910 in 1989 to $290 in 1999. Current per capita income is estimated at $170. Tajikistan's purchasing power parity is less than half of Uzbekistan's. As a result of the troubled economy, an estimated 700,000 men leave Tajikistan for Russia each year in search of work. According to some estimates, 60 percent of the male population between 16 and 30 works abroad.

Despite these difficulties, the Government has tried to respond to increasing rates of HIV infection and to mitigate the consequences of drug use. However, implementation of the National Program on HIV/AIDS and STIs has been slow. Relative to the threat that Tajikistan faces, current interventions to avert a generalized epidemic and coverage are largely inadequate. An encouraging sign has been the recent expansion of the NGO sector. There are currently more than a thousand NGOs registered in Tajikistan, although it is not clear how many of these are operational or funded. However NGOs are certainly active among populations vulnerable to heroin use.

Prevention and Control

Surveillance. Surveillance for HIV, STIs, and drug use continue to depend on compulsory notification/registration systems and outdated screening programs which persist from the Soviet era. Surveillance of drug use and dependency is carried out through the usual system of registration by clinicians of clinically confirmed cases in Narcology Services. There is a statutory obligation for physicians to maintain in this register newly identified individuals until they meet formal criteria for removal. Registration rates clearly underestimate the prevalence of drug use in the country. According to UNODC estimates (2003), 8 percent of all drug users are registered for treatment.

Adequate testing for HIV confirmation is only now becoming available in Tajikistan with GFATM funding. There are no firm plans for sentinel or behavioral surveillance of highly vulnerable groups (primarily testing for HIV and hepatitis markers) and linking these to prevalence and behavioral surveys among risk groups. There is an urgent need to ensure that sentinel and second-generation surveillance approaches be fully developed and extended as harm-reduction and prevention projects reach new geographic locations and risk sub-groups.

Routine HIV testing is only now becoming fully available in Tajikistan. However, there is standard surveillance carried out through laboratory testing of clinical and population groups as well as blood donations. Testing laboratories are mostly located in AIDS centers. With the help of GFATM funding, 13 labs received new lab equipment and necessary test kits, allowing the initiation of adequate testing/screening for HIV/AIDS. CDC has started providing technical assistance to establish sentinel surveillance in the country.

There is currently no sentinel surveillance for STIs. Better use could be made of existing data screening population segments to gain insights into HIV and STI prevalence rates. As in other countries in the region, surveillance of STIs is carried out through compulsory case notification by a network of 194 dermato-venereal specialists in 19 dispensaries, 36 general hospital departments, and 46 specialized rooms across the Republic. These services do not have any specific initiatives targeted at HIV risk groups such as CSWs and IDUs. Tajikistan continues to use a system of notification by clinicians of clinically confirmed cases of STIs as the primary means of STI surveillance.

Prevention among Vulnerable Groups. Rapid assessments suggest that there have been very large increases in the number of IDUs, CSWs, and migrants over the last 10 years in the country (Open Society Institute 2003). Income differentials and poverty create demand for and supply of CSWs, while the passage of drug trafficking routes carrying opiates through the country delivers a copious supply of cheap opium and heroin to fuel the epidemic of injecting drug use (Human Rights Watch 2003). Numbers of registered drug users continue to increase. Official Government estimates of 30,000 are almost certainly too low. There are an estimated 60,000 IDU and 5,000 CSW in the country and levels of risk behaviour appear high. Drug users are becoming younger, and there is a shift away from traditional opium injection to heroin injection, at least among registered users.

With the support of UNAIDS, international NGOs and local municipalities, 15 trust points for IDUs and one pilot project for CSWs have been set up. In addition, seven trust points (TP) for IDUs and six friendly clinics (FC) for CSWs were established in six cities around the country. However, these facilities only offer services to 400 IDUs (less than 1 percent of the estimated number of IDUs) and 100 CSWs (2 percent of the estimated number of CSWs). Trust points function as IDU harm-reduction projects but there is little information on the extent or coverage of their activities. Under the GFATM grant, the CCM plans to open 13 more trust points. However, these interventions cannot cover more than 10 percent of highly vulnerable groups.

The Government estimates that there are around 5,000 CSWs in the country. According to it, HIV seroprevalence among CSWs in Dushanbe is 1.1 percent. A detailed RAR assessment of CSWs in the country has been carried out within the framework of USAID's Drug Demand Reduction Project. A strong association between commercial sex work and injecting drug use was reported; and a tendency for economic need to be correlated with high risk sexual behavior. Migration is reported to be one of the key influences for women to get involved in sex work, especially for those within the lowest sectors of the sex industry. Not having residence permits greatly influences the living and working conditions of a migrant sex worker and is often found to lead to increased marginalization, isolation, dependency, and vulnerability to further exploitation and involvement in criminal activity. Sex workers were found to experience high levels of stigmatization, which drives them into drug use. Access to information on prevention methods and to health, social and advocacy services were low. Homosexual relationships are illegal in Tajikistan, but no further information on MSM was obtained.

Due to significant labor migration, which is estimated to be of about 620,000 people a year, out of which 84 percent migrate to Russia for a period of 8 to 9 months, Tajikistan faces a significant threat of having an increase in the share of heterosexual transmission. These fears are further supported by the following findings:

- Up to 80 percent of labor migrants are males;
- The largest share of male migrants can be divided into two main age groups: those who are 20–29 years-old and those who are 40–49 years-old, with 85 percent of them leaving wives and families behind;
- Most migrants engage in risky sexual behavior (having on average 2–3 different sex partners over a period of 6–9 months). Russia has a significant incidence of HIV, which puts at risk labor migrants and their wives.

AFEW has recently conducted a Rapid Assessment among male and female prison inmates within the context of the DDRP (OSI 2003). Although some of the findings are embargoed, the assessment conclusions are available. There was evidence of low levels of knowledge of HIV transmission routes especially through sex. Sexual activities reportedly occur but the degree is harder to determine given the apparent reluctance by prisoners to answer questions about it. The picture of prison sexual activity that can be drawn from the data is a complex and limited one. Only 7 percent of prisoners reported involvement in sexual relations while in prison; and a small percent among these had access to condoms. A significant proportion of inmates reported that they had previously used condoms during sexual intercourse. Tattooing in prison, in contrast to drugs and sex, is widespread. Close to half of the prisoners had tattoos and nearly a half of these had them made in prison. In terms of infectious diseases, tattooing may present an ideal transmission route for hepatitis as well as HIV. Injecting drugs in prison was less frequent. Of the sample who reported having ever injected, one third (33 percent) reported injecting drugs in prisons. Among prison injectors, 40 percent reported using previously used needles and/or syringes. The coverage of HIV testing is low (less than one third were tested for HIV). The prevalence of STI rates in prisons reflects the general trend of the epidemic process among the population. The number of STIs registered during the last 12 months (66 percent of those who ever had any STIs) reflects the coverage of testing and concern for health problems.

As 70 percent of Tajikistan's population is under 30 years-old, needs for youth IEC activities much exceed the resources available, mainly through UNICEF (2003). This agency has been providing assistance to a network of youth organizations, and supporting the school-based adolescent healthy lifestyle project and peer-to-peer HIV/AIDS education. UNFPA has been providing condoms for free distribution. Low level of knowledge on HIV/AIDS is an impediment to prevention. A UNAIDS rapid assessment among the population revealed that 60 percent does not know how HIV spreads or how to prevent its transmission. Awareness is particularly low in rural areas (OSI 2003). Among a representative sample of parents only 15 percent could name correctly the modes of HIV transmission, with women and Dushanbe residents scoring lower. Only 29 percent understood the relationship between HIV and injecting drug use.

Clinical and Laboratory Services. There are four Narcology Dispensaries, and 60 narcologists working in the dispensaries and a network of consultation centers throughout the country. Detoxification is the main clinical services that is provided and there is little social or psychological support. Currently the legislation requires that all patients are registered, although the chief narcologist has secured a change in instructions to allow provision of fully confidential services. The Narcology Service has not been involved in the GFATM grant application and implementation, and there is no replacement treatment component in the GFATM activity plan. Residential rehabilitation is available, but it is expensive in the private sector ($500).

Clinical and Laboratory services for HIV/AIDS are provided through the Republican Centre for AIDS Control and Prevention; regional AIDS Centers; and 24 HIV diagnostic laboratories. In addition to identifying and advocating for critical interventions, these centers provide HIV testing (including screening predetermined risk groups and blood donations), some counseling, treatment for HIV related diseases, and carry out epidemiological interviews with individuals testing positive for HIV. Until recently, national capacity to diagnose HIV/AIDS was very limited and consistent testing of blood supply was not guaranteed, with confirmatory testing being done only outside the country. With funds from GFATM and USAID grants, the country was planning to re-equip 70 percent of existing labs and procure test kits. So far the Government has managed to equip only about half of its laboratories with GFATM funding, and test kits were not procured in quantities needed for full-scale implementation of the National Program. The number of laboratories and structure of provision of laboratory services need to be reviewed. The AIDS structures have committed themselves to expanding VCT services, and there is a network of individuals trained in psychosocial counseling on HIV/AIDS. However, until recently tests have not been available and very few people have received VCT. Only palliative treatment is available—ARV therapy is still inaccessible for HIV/AIDS patients in Tajikistan (Basmakova and others 2003). However, WHO has provided $10,000 for development of clinical protocols for ARVT.

The technical base of the venereal diseases service has declined significantly over the last 10 years with decreasing Government funding. Reliable syphilis diagnostics are available but there are no reliable tests for chlamydia or gonorrhea infections in women. Essential STI drugs are available, at least in Dushanbe, but there are doubts about the availability of either tests or treatment at the periphery. Despite the lack of diagnostic equipment there has been no significant progress made towards adoption of syndromic management approaches recommended by WHO for such settings or management of STIs within generic health services. There has been an important and welcome shift from inpatient to outpatient management with the majority of cases now being treated as outpatients. Contact-tracing has also become more confidential and acceptable and links with police have weakened. Patients pay for all treatments: the average cost of treatment for syphilis, including consultations with specialists, is between $50 to $200.

The system of STI service provision continues to be broadly based on the old Soviet model. There are currently 19 dispensaries, 36 departments in general hospitals and 46 specialized rooms with 194 dermato-venereological specialists of different level. It was reported that more than 90 percent of syphilis cases are now treated in an outpatient setting with benzathine penicillin. There is a sufficient number of specialists skilled in the syndromic management approach for STIs. However, the Ministry of Health has not issued a relevant decree and the syndromic management approach has not been implemented so far. The private sector is poorly developed and its services are affordable only to wealthy clients.

Key Findings in Uzbekistan

In 2003 there were approximately 20,000 registered drug users (RDUs) of which around 11,000 were heroin users. GoU estimates that 50 percent of all drug users inject drugs. Cumulative cases of HIV increased rapidly from 2000 to reach 3,584 (15.0 per 100,000) by the end of 2003. There were 1,836 new HIV cases notified in 2003. The rate of annual notifications of new cases has increased rapidly since 2000 reaching 7.7 per 100,000 in 2003. The annual number of notified cases of syphilis increased from 1.8 per 100,000, to reach 47.3 per 100,000 in 1987 before falling to 21.8 per 10,000 in 2003.

Uzbekistan: Key Indicators at a glance (2003–2004)	
AIDS/HIV Deaths	155*
AIDS Cases—Cumulative	25
AIDS Cases—New	
HIV Cases—Cumulative	6,862*
HIV Cases—Cumulative/100,000	27.4*
Increase HIV—Cum. 2000–2003	16 fold
M:F Ratio HIV—Cumulative	
Proportion of HIV Cumulative among 20–29 yr. olds	
HIV Cumulative among IDU	
HIV Cases—New	2,016*
Proportion of New HIV acquired through IDU	59%*
HIV Cases—New/100,000	8*
M:F Ratio New Cases	4.4*
Highest Oblast new HIV rate	Tashkent City
New HIV /100,000 (all ages) in Highest Oblast	39.6
Estimated HIV Prevalence IDU	1.2%
Estimated HIV Prevalence Prisoners (males)	0.4%
Estimated prevalence in pregnant women	NA
Registered Drug Users	19,088
M:F Sex Ratio Drug Users	Estimated : 10:1
Registered IDU	9,500
Estimated IDU	65,000–90,000
Estimated HIV Preval. IDU	1.2%
Estimated CSW	20,000
Estimated MSM	NA

*Data for 2004

The Government has been steadily building its commitment and capacity to respond to HIV/AIDS. Most recently, the Government developed and approved the Strategic Program on Counteracting the HIV/AIDS Epidemic in the Republic of Uzbekistan for 2003–2006. However, there are also a number of negative factors within the risk environment. State structures concerned with prevention and treatment of infectious disease still play roles very much akin to policing infected individuals; and notably within the Dermatological and Venereal Diseases service, militia are still involved in capturing segments of the population (particularly CSW) and bringing these compulsorily into to the DVS. There is an attitude of closure and secrecy in relation to availability of official statistics describing HIV/STI and risk behaviors. The NGO sector exists; but is not flourishing or energetic in the same way as that in the Kyrgyz Republic. The Government has responded to the need for harm-reduction projects by issuing a decree to set up a large number of 'trust points' which should deliver VCT as well as advice and HR commodities; and does not significantly support NGOs in this work. These factors will need to be addressed if an effective large scale response is to be achieved. In addition low levels of knowledge on HIV/AIDS are likely to be an impediment to prevention.

Adequate testing for HIV with confirmation should become more widely available with delivery of the GFATM work program, allowing extension of VCT and trust point activity. Surveillance for HIV, STIs and drug use continue to depend on compulsory notification/ registration systems and outdated screening programs which persist from the Soviet era. CDC is developing sites for quality controlled laboratories including in Tashkent City, Tashkent Oblast, Andijan, Samarkand, and Termis (primarily testing for HIV and hepatitis markers), and linking these to prevalence and behavioral surveys among risk groups. There is an urgent need to ensure that sentinel and second-generation surveillance approaches continue to be supported and extended as new waves of harm-reduction and prevention projects reach new geographic locations and risk sub-groups. In particular, there is a need to review how the GFATM strengthened trust points may contribute to sentinel and second-generation surveillance. There is currently no sentinel surveillance for STIs. Better use could be made of existing data screening population segments to gain insights into HIV and STI prevalence rates.

HIV/AIDS and STI in Uzbekistan: Epidemiological Trends

Drug Use. In 2003, there were approximately 20,000 RDUs, out of which around 11,000 were heroin users. GoU estimates that 50 percent of all drug users inject drugs. According to official statistics between 1996 and 2000 there was a 270 percent increase in the number of people in the Republic suffering from drug addiction, and since 1991 there was an 800 percent increase. The largest increase in the number of drug addicts has been among persons aged 20–40. Persons from this age group accounted for 72 percent of the drug addicts that were registered for the first time in 2000. GoU estimates that there are 65–90,000 drug users in the country, with 17–22,000 of them living in Tashkent and 15–22,000 in Samarkand (Uzbek CCM 2003). These estimates are broadly consistent with UNODC estimates (2003).

HIV/AIDS. Cumulative cases increased rapidly in the past few years reaching 3,584 (15.0 per 100,000) by the end of 2003. New cases have also continued to rapidly increase since 2000 reaching 7.7 per 100,000 in 2003. The male:female ratio in 2002 was 4:2. The age distribution analysis for males tested HIV positive shows that the overwhelming majority is between 25 and 40 years-old. A fairly large share (16 percent) of men is between 15 and 24. Among women, 23 percent of the 188 cases notified in 2002 were among 15 to 24 year-olds and 65 percent among 25 to 40 year-olds.

In the GFATM application, the Government reports that 65 percent of HIV infections was through drug injections. According to the 2001 results of sentinel surveillance in Tashkent, HIV prevalence among drug users was 45 percent (Uzbek CCM 2003). GoU official statistics suggest HIV prevalence rates of 1.2 percent among 18,000 IDUs; and

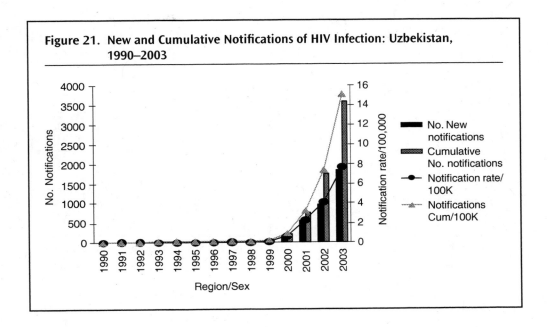

Figure 21. New and Cumulative Notifications of HIV Infection: Uzbekistan, 1990–2003

0.4 percent among 65,000 prisoners. It has not been possible to obtain confirmation of these figures or throw light on the methods used in arriving at them.

As Figure 21 shows, there has been a sharp rise in the number of cumulative cases between 2000 and 2003. The geographical distribution of the number of notifications of new cases shows that Tashkent has the highest number of HIV positive individuals (Figure 22).

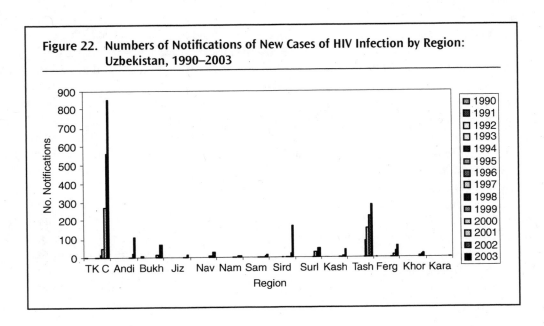

Figure 22. Numbers of Notifications of New Cases of HIV Infection by Region: Uzbekistan, 1990–2003

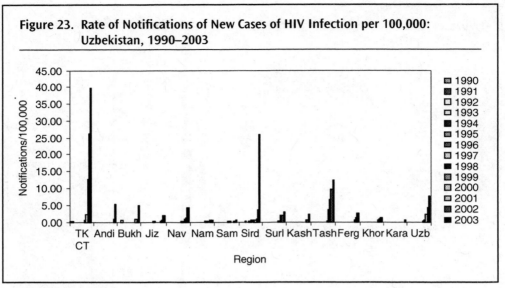

Figure 23. Rate of Notifications of New Cases of HIV Infection per 100,000: Uzbekistan, 1990–2003

Source: MoH Uzbekistan.

As Figure 23 shows, the gap between the capital and the rest of the country becomes smaller when rates are considered.

Patterns almost certainly primarily reflect testing (although numbers of tests carried out year on year in different regions were not obtained). The notification rate in Tashkent in 2003 reached 40 per 100,000 and in Sirdaryo 26/100,000. The cumulative notification rate for men aged 15 to 24 in Tashkent is estimated to be around 250 per 100,000 or 0.25 percent.

Annual numbers of notified cases of syphilis increased from 363 (1.8 per 100,000) to 11,050 (47 per 100,000) in 1997 then declined and stabilized below 10 per 100,000 during 2000–2003. The size of the syphilis epidemic in Uzbekistan is similar to that in Turkmenistan; but smaller than those in the Kyrgyz Republic and Kazakhstan. It is not clear whether this lower prevalence and the decline since 1997 reflect a real decline in incidence or changes in service accessibility or accuracy in notification. It can be seen that the age distribution for men and women is very similar, and that men and women over 30 have higher rates of syphilis. The number of notifications of new cases of syphilis in different regions of Uzbekistan between 1990 and 2003 are shown in Figure 24; and the corresponding rate per 100,000 population in Figure 25.

The figures show a very rapid rise in syphilis occurrence in the early 1990s, peaking around 1996–98 in all regions but the largest number of cases was observed in Tashkent and Fergana. The data suggest the epidemic occurred across the country; but rates suggest a concentration in Syrdario, Navoi, and Fergana. In 1996, in Tashkent City the overall notification rate exceeded 120 per 100,000 population. It seems likely that the decline in the late 1990s represents a combination of a real decline in the incidence of syphilis, together with a decrease in the proportion of registered cases due to changing patterns of clinical

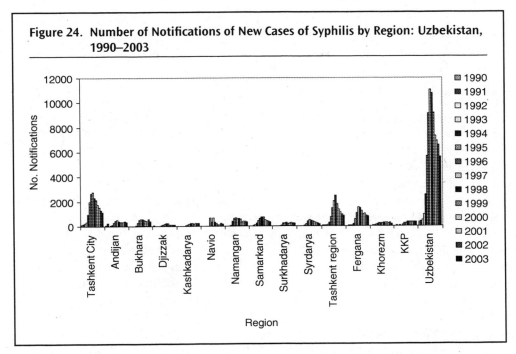

Figure 24.   Number of Notifications of New Cases of Syphilis by Region: Uzbekistan, 1990–2003

Source: MoH Uzbekistan.

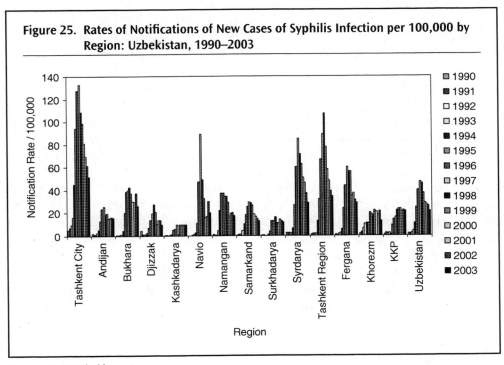

Figure 25.   Rates of Notifications of New Cases of Syphilis Infection per 100,000 by Region: Uzbekistan, 1990–2003

Source: MoH Uzbekistan.

care and notification rates. The dermatovenereology service in Tashkent reported finding one case of syphilis among 1,000 women screened in 2003.

Risk Behavior and Environment

Uzbekistan is a dry, landlocked country with 11 percent of its territory consisting of intensely cultivated, irrigated river valleys. More than 60 percent of its population lives in densely populated rural communities. Uzbekistan is now the world's second-largest cotton exporter, a large producer of gold and oil, and a regionally significant producer of chemicals and machinery. Following independence in December 1991, the government sought to prop up its Soviet-style command economy with subsidies and tight controls on production and prices. Uzbekistan responded to the negative external conditions generated by the Asian and Russian financial crises by emphasizing import substitute industrialization and by tightening export and currency controls within its already largely closed economy. A growing debt burden, persistent inflation, and a poor business climate led to disappointing growth in 2001–02. The government, while aware of the need to improve the investment climate, sponsors measures that often increase, not decrease the government's control over business decisions. A sharp increase in the inequality of income distribution has hurt the lower ranks of society since independence.[18] GNP in 2002 was estimated at $2,500 growing at 3 percent annually.

Poverty remains a serious problem in Uzbekistan: 27.5 percent of the population or 6.8 million people were considered as being poor in 2000/01 with one third of them (>2 million) considered as being extremely poor. Poverty is predominantly a rural phenomenon; 62 percent of the population lives in rural areas. Participation in secondary schooling has declined sharply. After independence, the proportion of adolescents between the ages of 15–18 entering high school fell by 24 percent to 2000 (Bernard and others 2001).

Like its neighbors Uzbekistan is seeing an explosion in injecting drug use and commercial sex work with the development of local markets for opiates trafficked from Afghanistan, since the early 1990s. This explosion, combined with an increase in STIs and economic migration, including shuttle migration to high HIV prevalence areas in CIS and elsewhere, create a serious threat of a major HIV epidemic initially concentrated among IDUs but with a potential to rapidly spread through sexual transmission to the general population.

Rapid assessments suggests that there have been very large increases in the number of IDUs, CSWs, and migrants over the last 10 years. Income differentials and poverty create demand for and supply of CSWs; while the passage of drug trafficking routes carrying opiates through the country delivers a copious supply of cheap opium and heroin to fuel the epidemic of injecting drug use. Hostile and dishonest police behavior in relation to CSWs and IDUs certainly occurs throughout the country, driving CSWs and IDUs into patterns of behavior associated with very high risks of HIV transmission (Human Rights Watch 2003). High unemployment rates drive high levels of migration within and outside the country, including to destinations with higher background prevalence of HIV infection. This is likely to be continuously seeding infection into the population. A decline in

---

18. This information is available at http://www.theodora.com/wfb2003/uzbekistan/uzbekistan_economy.html

social support services and participation in education as well as unemployment leaves young people increasingly vulnerable to HIV risk behaviors and infection.

GoU has been steadily building its commitment and capacity to respond to HIV/AIDS. Most recently, the Government developed and approved the Strategic Program on Counteracting the HIV/AIDS Epidemic in the Republic of Uzbekistan for 2003–2006. Uzbekistan has a general information, education and communications (IEC) strategy on HIV/AIDS, which includes specific initiatives for vulnerable groups. A letter on accelerated access to ARV drugs was signed by the Minister of Health and sent to WHO and UNAIDS.

However, there are also a number of negative factors within the risk environment. State structures concerned with the prevention and treatment of infectious disease still play roles very much akin to policing infected individuals; and notably within the Dermatovenereology service, police is still involved in capturing segments of the population (particularly CSW) and compulsorily bringing them to the DVS. There is an attitude of closure and secrecy in relation to availability of official statistics describing HIV/STI and risk behaviors. The NGO sector exists, but it is not flourishing or as energetic as that in the Kyrgyz Republic. The Government has responded to the need for harm-reduction projects by issuing a decree to set up a large number of "trust points" which should deliver VCT as well as advice and HR commodities. However, it does not significantly support NGOs in this work. These factors will need to be addressed if an effective scaled-up response is to be achieved. In addition low levels of knowledge on HIV/AIDS are likely to be an impediment to prevention.

The GoUs application to the GFATM states "The most significant programmatic gap is the lack of prevention initiatives for the vulnerable populations that are most at-risk of contracting HIV/AIDS (Uzbek CCM 2003). Currently, the coverage of prevention programs for IDUs, CSWs, MSM, and prisoners is less than 1 percent for each group. In addition, IDUs, CSWs, and MSM have a severely limited access to health services, including STI diagnosis and treatment, due to stigma and discrimination. As most PLWHAs are from one of these vulnerable groups, they face an even higher level of stigma and discrimination.

According to one of the studies carried out in Uzbekistan, since 1995, there has been a sharp increase in drug addiction.[19] Heroin addiction is currently the main factor driving the increase in the number of drug addicts. There is a predominance of persons aged 25 to 35 among registered drug users. Between 1996 and 2000, there was a nine-fold increase in the number of drug addicts undergoing treatment in drug treatment centers. There has been a general increase in the rates of drug-related crime. In the middle of the 1990s heroin began to replace traditional drugs, such as opium and hash (marijuana), on the illicit drugs market. This has brought about a transformation in the existing pattern of drug use and heroin is now the drug that is most commonly used (including prisons), followed by opium and cannabis. It is administered predominantly through injection, with people first using the drug in the company of friends and primarily because they want to experience new sensations.

Among drug addicts in Tashkent there is a predominance of persons with either incomplete or complete secondary education, whereas in the Samarkand region, there is a

---

19. 'Qalb Sadosi' Social Foundation (a non-governmental not-for-profit organisation) recently carried out a RAR of drug use in the country with the approval of GoU; financial and technical assistance from UNODC, and with the support and assistance of the National Drug Control Centre.

predominance of persons with secondary or just primary education. The majority of drug addicts are either unemployed or work only occasionally. Research also indicates very high risk behaviors among IDUs, including regular sharing of needles and syringes and the use of human blood in the preparation of drug solutions (Uzbek CCM 2003). The level of knowledge among drug addicts about risk factors associated with HIV infection is extremely low. About half of the respondents who inject drugs (IDUs) reported to have had sexual contacts with other IDUs. Moreover, they started to have sexual contacts more frequently after having started injecting drugs. Only a small percentage use condoms during penetrative sex, either with permanent or casual sexual partners. Almost half of surveyed IDUs had paid for sex in the last 12 months. IDUs in general are not aware of the HIV status of their sexual partners. It was estimated by the UNDP office that less than 10 percent of IDUs in Uzbekistan are female and that 40 to 50 percent of them engage in commercial sex (Dallabetta and Gavrilin 2001). Half of IDUs have had STIs.

The number of CSWs operating in Uzbekistan is not well estimated. In 2000, it was estimated that 5,000 CSWs were working in Tashkent, out of which 30 to 40 percent were IDUs (Dehne and Kobyscha 2000). Information obtained from the Tashkent Derma-tovenereology service suggested that at least 3,000 CSWs were known to city police and were brought to the DVS on a regular basis for STI screening. On the basis of these findings, previously published overall estimates of 20,000 CSWs in the country as a whole seem reasonable. Evidence suggests that although condoms are readily available from kiosks, the majority of CSW do not use condoms with clients (Godinho and others 2004). Findings from the 1997 UNAIDS assessment may now be out of date, but they point to certain issues which may still be important. First, the role of police in securing mandatory HIV and STD testing, and confining those infected, deters CSW from accessing the state run HIV and STD services. Most are likely to seek care from private physicians. Second, the majority of clients refuse to use condoms, and when pimps are involved in the negotiation of price, the "contract" does not specify condom use. Third, CSWs routinely pay "protection" money to police and/or others who control the sex industry and provide free sexual services to them.

There are undoubtedly a large number of men who have sex with men in Uzbekistan, but this risk group is the most stigmatized and least understood. Social taboos concerning homosexuality have played a large part in marginalizing MSM. Most men in this group are forced to hide their sexual behavior out of fear of persecution and prosecution, making it difficult for them to obtain information on issues such as safe sex and HIV/AIDS (Population Services International 2001).

There is considerable migration of Uzbek populations, both external and internal, the latter being especially from rural areas to big cities. Migrant groups are likely to be important for HIV spread, but they are not recognized to be at-risk groups within the Government's HIV/AIDS strategy.

According to official statistics from the Uzbek Ministry of Interior, 11.7 percent of prisoners in 2000 were jailed for a drug-related crime (OSI 2003). The Ministry of Interior has its own health care department, which is responsible for the health of inmates, disease surveillance and epidemic control in detention facilities. There are 53 prisons in total with 47,000 inmates. Around 12,200 are leaving and entering the prisons each year. The HIV epidemic in prisons is growing. The first case of HIV in prisons was registered in 1998, but already in 1999, there were 19 cases, and by 2002, around 200.

Prevention and Control

Surveillance. Routine HIV surveillance is carried out through health service structures in testing laboratories located mostly in the AIDS centers. The samples originate from clinical and population groups and blood donations. Tested groups include: registered drug users, patients with STI diagnoses, and pregnant women. Testing is irregular—it varies in particular with test availability, although laboratory infrastructure is being reinforced with support from CDC, GFATM grant, and Bank-financed Uzbek Health II Project. Positive screening tests are required to be confirmed by Western Blot. Identified HIV infected persons are invited to attend clinical services where an epidemiological interview is conducted to establish key demographic variables and likely route of transmission. Standard notifications forms and statistical summaries cascade completed information on HIV positive individuals to the center.

Uzbekistan continues to use a system of notification by clinician of clinically confirmed cases of sexually transmitted infection as the primary means of STI surveillance. There is a statutory obligation for physicians to notify each person newly identified as being infected with STIs (syphilis and gonorrhea) that requires registration. The infection can be identified either through passive diagnosis in patients presenting to clinical services, or through active case finding in previous sexual contacts of newly detected cases. During the Soviet period this system probably identified the majority of diagnosed cases of syphilis. However, since 1990 it is very likely that there has been a decline in the accuracy of notification rates as a result of an increasing tendency among patients to use paid, anonymous services obtained in the public or private sector, lack of funding for the Dermatovenereology and STI structures, and limited availability of sensitive and specific diagnostic tests. Strict case definitions for reporting which do not reflect the fact that, in reality, cases may be syndromically diagnosed and managed further complicate the issue of reporting.

Surveillance of drug use and dependency is carried out by a system of registration by clinicians of clinically confirmed cases in Narcology Services. There is a statutory obligation for physicians to keep in this register all newly identified individuals until they meet formal criteria for removal. Registration rates clearly underestimate the prevalence of drug use in the country, but UNODC estimates (2003) that as many as 18 percent of all drug users may be registered.

With the support of CDC and USAID, the country is moving towards adoption of sentinel surveillance within the framework of Second-Generation HIV Surveillance recommended by WHO/UNAIDS (2000). Current sites that are under development include Tashkent City, Tashkent Oblast, Andijan, Samarkand, and Termis. The focus is on supporting development of laboratory capacity for HIV and hepatitis testing and quality control systems. Training as well as systematic evaluation of the sensitivity and specificity of diagnostics produced in the region are being conducted. In addition, in collaboration with outreach and harm-reduction projects prevalence surveys linked to behavioral surveys are being carried out among risk groups.

Prevention among Vulnerable Groups. Over the past 2–3 years the GoU has ordered the establishment of 230 trust points (TPs) financed from central and local budgets and placed within the public health care facilities. These TPs are intended to deliver harm-reduction activities to GAR, including needle exchange, condom supply, social and legal counseling, and some medical services. Each TP employs one doctor, one nurse and one other support staff member. However, due to lack of adequate human and financial resources needle exchange is in effect the only service offered by TPs. During 2002, TPs only exchanged 1 million syringes, which amounts to about 12 syringes per day per facility. Moreover, most TPs are placed within public provider institutions, which prevents IDUs from seeking care from them. IDUs largely do not trust them and do not seek care from government-run TPs.

To improve quality of services offered by trust points significant investments are required for: a) human resource development and b) infrastructure upgrades. Current GoU regulations do not have flexibility to establish more TPs in those areas where drug use is more prevalent. Rather regulations mandate to establish one TP for every 50,000 population (standard Soviet type input based financing of service provision). Such mandates do not take into account local needs and are not demand driven. Therefore GoU TPs are not currently a viable front-line service for the work with high-risk groups. TPs opened and operated by local and international NGOs offer services that are more acceptable and have better locations. NGOs try to employ volunteers and use peer-to-peer approach. The relative effectiveness of these TPs is likely to be much higher when compared to government ones.

In Tashkent, a Soros funded NGO, SABO, started working with CSWs in 1999. The main activities include education on reproductive health and STIs, provide legal consultation and operate a telephone hotline. To date, the total number of 200 CSWs have sought counseling from this NGO. Of these, 60 percent were Russian and 40 percent of other nationalities. Twenty percent of women in this group have children. The NGO is noting a trend towards younger CSWs with many of them coming to the city from rural areas. It also reports that police and clients abuse CSWs. In addition, the Tashkent City Dermatovenereology Service reported that local police brings in about 3,000 women whom they have identified as CSWs for STI screening, sometimes several times per year.

Traditionally little emphasis has been placed on the prevention of STIs through education and health promotion initiatives, although case-finding and contact-tracing have been assiduously carried out. Condoms are usually not offered at dermatovenereology clinics or hospital services either for free or for a fee.

Clinical and Laboratory Services. There are 18 Narcology Dispensaries with 500 narcologists and a network of consultation centers (specialized rooms) throughout the country. Detoxification is the main clinical service that is provided with little social or psychological support. Current legislation requires for all patients to register. Residential rehabilitation is available but it is in the private sector and expensive. However, innovative changes in what is otherwise a standard Soviet model of narcology services are gradually taking place. The Narcology Dispensary in Tashkent is operating a needle exchange point. It has also diversified its staff and service base with the aim of introducing extended psychological therapies and rehabilitation programs, as well as managing an increasing number of patients on an outpatient basis. In addition, there has been an increasing recognition of the need to secure the cooperation from police, hence, a number of trainings have been carried out for local police officers. A Swiss funded project on HR, including outreach and MST, has been implemented and has influenced the proposals to extend MST within the GFATM application.

Clinical and Laboratory services for HIV/AIDS are provided through the Republican Centre for AIDS Control and Prevention and its network of 14 associated regional AIDS Centers and 92 HIV diagnostic laboratories. These centers aim at providing HIV testing (including screening predetermined risk groups as well as blood donations), some counseling, treatment for HIV related disease, as well as carrying out epidemiological interviews with individuals testing positive for HIV/AIDS. They also identify and advocate for critical interventions. However, in reality, financial and human resource constraints severely restrict the activities of these centers.

The quality of diagnostic testing equipment in these facilities is poor. While the recent GFATM grant and Bank-financed Health II Project will upgrade a number of laboratories, the Republican AIDS Centre wishes to upgrade all 92 laboratories. However, a careful review is needed of the overall provision of HIV testing services to ensure their cost-effectiveness and, when possible, economies of scale. The AIDS structures have committed themselves to expanding VCT services and there is a network of individuals trained in psychological and social counseling on HIV/AIDS. However, until recently tests have been rarely available and very few people have received VCT. Only palliative treatment is available and there is little use of ARVs, at least in the public sector (Uzbek CCM 2003).

STI services continue to be provided through Dermatovenereology Service structures and these have been slow to modernize, or transform into an effective, public health service. There are ten dispensaries distributed across the country and 217 specialized rooms in area hospitals. In order to receive affordable treatment within DV structures one still needs to have identification documents and registration, although there are anonymous services but they are not free and tend to be expensive. All outpatient treatment is to be paid at full cost. Forty percent of cases of syphilis are still managed as inpatients, with multiple daily injections of penicillin during a 16 day stay. STI drugs can be obtained in major towns but their availability in the periphery is uncertain and is most likely to be limited. Funding from GoU probably represents no more than 20 percent of the total resources flowing to the DVS; the remainder comes from out-of-pocket payments on the part of patients. Active case-finding through screening occupational and clinical groups continues but is declining. Contact-tracing approaches still conform to the old Soviet model, with police supported "rapid response groups" forcibly bringing identified contacts to DV services for screening and treatment. Around 3,000 CSWs known to the police are brought in this manner each year in Tashkent City alone. Syphilis diagnostic tests are available in central laboratories, but availability of such testing at the periphery seems to be restricted.

Despite its slow modernization the system shows some promising signs. The Tashkent City DVS in collaboration with the Republican AIDS Center is in the process of setting up a new anonymous sexual health service facility for CSWs in the city. In addition, the New HIV Strategic Program emphasizes the need for the introduction of syndromic treatment, however, as in other countries, these innovations are likely to be resisted by dermatovenereologists. If current plans within GFATM to deliver STI services through trust points are implemented, then this could prove to be a major drive for innovation within STI services generally.

The Economic Consequences of HIV in Central Asia: Simulation Model Approach

This study suggests that HIV in Central Asia is likely to have a far-reaching impact on the economic development of the region. A slowdown in GDP growth and losses in GDP level may be accompanied by losses in effective labor supply, which would be worsened by negative population growth in some countries. The study also indicates that, at current prices, the costs of HIV treatment will not be sustainable by the public budget if the epidemic is not prevented, and/or treatment costs are not cut dramatically. As a policy implication, decisionmakers are advised to launch prevention programs, especially among highly vulnerable groups. Injecting drug users (IDU) are currently the group most at risk and, therefore, the most risky channel for HIV transmission. Preventing the spread of HIV among IDU is advisable to prevent subsequent sexual transmission to vulnerable groups that do not inject drugs.

Design of the Simulation Model and the User Interface

This study follows an interactive simulation approach to depict recent HIV/AIDS developments in the selected Central Asia countries (currently Kazakhstan, Kyrgyz Republic, and Uzbekistan) and predict the economic consequences of the HIV/AIDS epidemic in the region, under various scenarios.

The computer model designed to mimic HIV/AIDS and economic developments connects input parameters and output variables. It has been successfully probed to predict the economic consequences of HIV/AIDS in Russia (used hereafter as a reference point; Ruhl and others 2003). Ten output variables display the human, economic and fiscal costs of HIV/AIDS. A total of 26 input parameters need to be determined to derive these results.

It is one of the key features of the model to leave maximum discretion to the user, who is free to determine and change the 17 input parameters most relevant for modeling the diffusion of HIV, and the costs and results of policies designed to minimize the spread of HIV. Wherever applicable, the data used to calculate the economic model are the same as the data used by the official authorities that provide the economic and budget forecast. The parameters not accessible to manipulation are either historical data important in defining the model's initial conditions (that is, the size of the population and the number of drug users in 2003); or specifications of the underlying economic model calculated to derive the budget and official government forecasts (the parameters of the production function, the depreciation rate); or, where official government estimates do not exist, estimates made closely in line with the latter and based on standard empirical resources (international interest rate, labor productivity of drug users, infected non-drug users, and non-infected non-drug users, and the saving rate of the HIV positive population).[20]

The parameters open to manipulation by the user encompass four main groups:

- Determinants of the spread of HIV across the population, i.e. the speed of transmission among intravenous drug users, from drug users to non-drug users, and among non-drug users, as well as the growth rate of intravenous drug users and the "multiplier" used to translate registered HIV positive cases into the actual number.[21]
- Assumptions about antiretroviral and medical treatment costs and coverage, which are important to estimate the costs and benefits of policies designed to minimize the economic and fiscal consequences of HIV, in effect the monthly costs of antiretroviral drug treatment, the share of recipients of free antiretroviral medication among the infected population, the cost of other medical care, including hospitalization, and the share of recipients who receive this treatment free of charge (financed by the budget), as well as the budgetary costs of eventual prevention programs.
- Economic variables important in estimating the economic consequences of HIV, such as the share of the labor force, the tax rate (imposed on households), the share of government revenues used for public investment, minimum budgetary expenditures, the share of after-tax income which is saved, and the international and domestic interest rates.
- Demographic indicators, *i.e.* the rate of growth of the population.

The outputs of the simulation model specify the human, economic and fiscal costs, along with demographic consequences of HIV pandemic, that is:

- Mortality rates as well as (cumulative) HIV infections,
- GDP and GDP growth,

---

20. In addition, the model assumes that the total number of drug users will never exceed 15 percent of the total population and the total number of HIV positive people will never exceed 60 percent. These assumptions were suggested by the Russian AIDS Center. Both of these assumptions slow down the diffusion of drug use and HIV infections, respectively.

21. Special emphasis is given to IDU because in the early stages of HIV epidemic this risk group quantitatively—and qualitatively—is most affected by the disease, and later on channels HIV to the rest of population through sexual contacts.

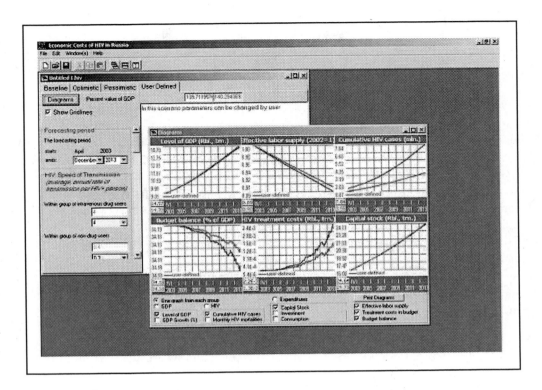

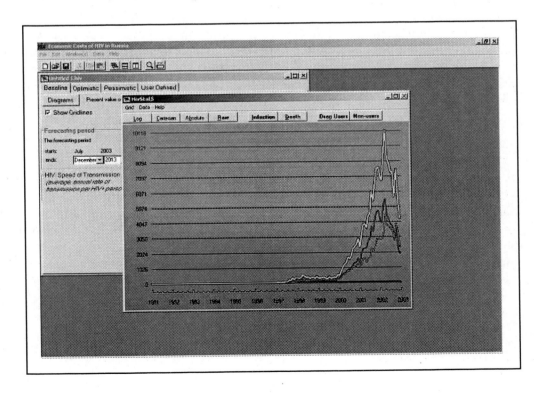

■ The value of the physical capital stock, of investment and consumption over time,
■ Budgetary treatment costs,
■ The budget balance, and
■ The effective, productivity adjusted, labor supply.

The first screenshot above exemplifies an output of the model. Also, the user has an option to see the history of HIV development. The past profiles of cumulative and monthly mortalities and HIV registered cases by source of infection can be plotted in absolute, Cartesian, or logarithmic coordinated. The second screenshot above provides an example.

The model can be setup in either English or Russian language. In the beginning of the computer simulation session, the user chooses a country from the list of suggested countries. This list is not fixed and can be extended (provided the appropriate country data is available). Currently, the covered countries include Kazakhstan, the Kyrgyz Republic, Uzbekistan, and Russia as a reference point.

The Economic Model

Production of Output. The underlying economic model is a simple and robust neoclassical model where output is a function of labor and capital, and where at any point in time $t = 1, 2, 3, \ldots$ the production function is of Cobb-Douglas type:

$$Y_t = A_t \cdot K_t^{\alpha} \cdot K_t^{\beta}$$

where K_t denotes capital and L_t effective labor supply in period t, and A_t is the total factor productivity (TFP). Both, capital and effective labor input are normalized to 1 at the beginning of the forecasting period. Following the estimates provided by IMF, the values of α and β are values of $\alpha = 0.3$ and $\beta = 0.7$ (Saavalainen and others 2003). The TFP, according to standard analysis of a transition country's production possibilities curve, is assumed to stay at 4 percent for three-five years and gradually decline later (Havrylyshin and others 1999 or Economic Expert Group estimates in Russia). This function, along with values of α and β, is not open to manipulation by the user.

The growth rate of output is given by: $\dot{Y}_t = \dfrac{Y_t - Y_{t-1}}{Y_{t-1}}, \; t = 1, 2, 3, \ldots$

Population Growth and Labor Supply. The growth rate of the population, n, is exogenous and can be changed by the user to reflect various scenarios of demographic development. Similarly, the active labor force (as a percentage of the total population) remains constant over the forecasting period, and the user can change the numerical value of this parameter. At each point in time, the total population is composed of four groups:

■ HIV—negative intravenous drug users (IDUs)
■ HIV—positive IDUs
■ HIV—negative non-IDUs, and
■ HIV—positive non-IDUs, denoted as N_t^{D-}, N_t^{D+}, N_t^{nonD+}, N_t^{nonD-}, respectively.

N^+ and N^- stand for the cumulative number of HIV-positive and HIV-negative people, and N^D and N^{nonD} denote the cumulative number of IDUs and non-IDUs, respectively, and N^{total} the entire population. The growth rate of the group of intravenous drug users, d, is estimated from the existing data and can be defined or changed by the user of the simulation program, subject to the limitation that no more than 15 percent of the population can become drug users at any point in time:[22]

$$N_t^D = N_{t-1}^D + d \cdot (0.15 \cdot N_{t-1}^{total} - N_{t-1}^D) - M_{t-1}^D \qquad (1)$$

where M_t^p is the mortality of drug users.

In line with international medical evidence, the share of HIV positive persons in the total population (that is, not only within the active work force) in this model has a negative impact on the productivity of labor. Anxiety, the need to provide home care, increased sick leave, and so forth will all negatively effect the active labor supply.[23] The model thus assumes lower productivity for the HIV infected segment of the population.[24]

However, HIV and AIDS can affect intravenous drug users as well as non-drug users. The economic model therefore discriminates between three groups. The highest productivity of labor is assigned to the non-HIV positive group of non-drug users, whereas the group of HIV positive non-IDUs has a lower productivity, and the lowest productivity level is assigned to the group of intravenous drug users, no matter whether HIV infected or not. These three productivity levels of IDU, HIV positive non-IDU and HIV negative non-IDU are denoted as p_1, p_2, and p_3 and set equal to 0.5, 0.87 and 1.0, respectively.

Total population

$$N_t^{total} = N_t^{D-} + N_t^{D+} + N_t^{nonD-} + N_t^{nonD+}, \qquad (2)$$

where m denotes the active labor force as a percentage of total population. Adjusted for productivity levels, the effective labor supply at time t, L_t, becomes the weighted average

$$L_t = p_1 \cdot m \cdot N_t^D + p_2 \cdot m \cdot N_t^{nonD+} + p_3 \cdot m \cdot N_t^{nonD-}. \qquad (3)$$

HIV adversely affects the effective labor supply through an increase in the percentage of HIV positive workers, and through increasing mortalities due to HIV/AIDS. To measure the pace and scope of spread of HIV, we distinguish between three different transmission rates of the disease:

- ▨ π_1 = HIV transmission within the group of intravenous drug users,
- ▨ π_2 = from intravenous drug users to non-drug users,[25]
- ▨ π_3 = within the group of non-drug users.

---

22. This assumption was suggested by the AIDS Center in Russia, based on international experience.

23. This diversion of resources occurs despite the fact that HIV positive people are theoretically capable of maintaining a full workload in the earlier stages of development of HIV.

24. Wherever applicable, while calibrating the model epidemiological data provided by the Russian AIDS Centre in Moscow, were used.

25. In general, this parameter may be used to capture the rate of transmission of HIV to low/medium risk group from any high-risk group, not necessarily IDU. For instance, it was observed in China that 40 percent of homosexuals are married and 25 percent have female sexual partners.

In different scenarios, the transmission rate among drug users is 2 for the optimistic and 4 for the pessimistic case (that is, one intravenous drug user is estimated to infect 2 or 4 other drug users per year). The transmission rate among non-drug users, in line with international estimates, has been set at 0.3 and 0.4, respectively. The rate with which HIV is transmitted from drug users to non-drug users has been kept at this same level.

The estimation of actual number of HIV cases is based on the statistics on registered cases by source of infection that has been provided by national AIDS Centers. The multiplier, μ, determines the relationship between registered and actual HIV infected persons (with actual cases equal to registered HIV positive cases times the multiplier). For each country, there are brackets for μ to depict optimistic and pessimistic scenario.

As suggested by the Russian AIDS Centre, the total number of HIV infected cannot exceed 60 percent of the total population. To evaluate the number of death cases in each period in time, we follow the international practice and assume that the life expectancy of HIV positive people starting from the moment of infection follows a Weibull distribution, with median 12 years.[26]

In our model, in each period the number of mortality cases is a sum of expected death cases of HIV positive IDU and HIV positive non-IDU in the absence of antiretroviral treatment, $M_t = M_t^{D-} + M_t^{nonD}$. If the share ($c_1$) of HIV positive drug users and non drug users receives preventive antiretroviral medication, then the mortality of HIV positive declines accordingly:[27]

$$M_t = (1-c_1) \cdot (M_t^{D-} + M_t^{nonD+}) \tag{4}$$

Given the transmission rates, the dynamics of the number of HIV positive IDU and non-IDU thus is depicted as follows:

$$N_t^{nonD+} = N_{t-1}^{nonD+} + \pi_3 \cdot (N_{t-1}^{nonD+}/N_{t-1}^{total}) + L_{t-1}^{nonD-} + \pi_2 \cdot (N_{t-1}^{D+}/N_{t-1}^{total}) \cdot N_{t-1}^{nonD-} - N_{t-1}^{nonD+},$$

$$N_t^{D+} = N_{t-1}^{D+} + \pi_1 \cdot (N_{t-1}^{D+}/N_{t-1}^{total}) \cdot L_{t-1}^{D-} - M_{t-1}^{D-}. \tag{5}$$

Formation of Physical Capital. The growth rate of capital is by gross investment net of depreciation:

$$K_t = K_{t-1}(1-\delta) + I_{t-1} \tag{6}$$

where the depreciation rate is parameterized as ($\delta = 0.05$, in line with IMF and WB estimates.

Investment consists of public (government) and private investment. Investment equals savings; government as well as household consumption becomes the residual of aggregate output:

$$I_t = I_{t-1}^{private} + I_{t-1}^{public}$$
$$I_t = S_t \tag{7}$$
$$Y_t = C_t + S_t$$

---

26. Existing statistics reveal that about 50 percent of HIV positive die in 12 years, and at least 95 percent die within 20 years after being infected, thus the estimates for mean and variance figures. However, the number 95 percent is believed by many experts to be underreported because not all patients are monitored for the entire 20 years period.

27. According to UNAIDS, regular intake of antiretroviral drugs prevents development of AIDS for an unlimited period of time.

The tax rate τ is defined by the user. As a percentage of output, private investments are defined as follows:

$$I_t^{private} = S_t^{effective\_private} + I_{t-1}^{public} \cdot (1-\tau) \cdot Y_t \tag{8}$$

The effective rate of private investment, $S_t^{effective\_private}$, is defined as the weighted average of the investment rates of HIV negative and HIV positive non-IDU (the group of IDUs is assumed not to make any savings/investment). Private savings (investment) of the group of non infected non-IDUs, s^{pr}, can be defined by the user, whereas infected non-IDUs are estimated to save, on average, about 50 percent less (with the value of the corrective multiplier, $s^+ = 0.5$):

$$s_t^{effective\_private} = \frac{(s^{pr} \cdot L_t^{nonD-} + s^{pr} \cdot s^+ \cdot L_t^{nonD+})}{(L_t^{nonD-} + L_t^{nonD+})} \tag{9}$$

As a percentage of output, public investments are defined as

$$I_t^{public} = S^{public} \cdot \max(0, CBS_t) \tag{10}$$

Here s^{public} denotes the share of public investment, and current budget surplus, CBS_t, is defined to be the tax revenues, $\tau \cdot Y_t$, net of antiretroviral costs, other medical treatment costs, debt payment and minimum public expenditures that have to be maintained (MPE_t), all of which are user defined parameters.

The Budget. The government has consumption and investment expenditures, and finances these expenditures by a tax on output. It faces an intertemporal budget constraint (is allowed to run a deficit). If taxes are raised to finance this deficit, household savings and therefore aggregate investment is affected immediately: if the deficit is run to finance consumption expenditures (such as medical treatments or drugs), aggregate investment will decline. The interest rate on domestic debt, i, can be set above, below, or equal to the exogenous discount rate, r, by the user of the simulation program.

Households do not borrow. If government expenditures for medical treatment increase, other government consumption and government investment have to be cut first, but at most down to the minimum public expenditure level, if such a level has been defined. For additional expenditures, the government will have to run a deficit. The budget level, B, is

$$B_t = \tau \cdot Y_t - I_t^{public} - (1+i) \cdot D_{t-1} - MPE_t - (c_1 \cdot RC + c_2 \cdot MC) \cdot (N^{D+} + N^{nonD+}). \tag{11}$$

Here c_1 denotes the percentage of HIV positive receivers of free, preventive (antiretroviral) medication, RC is the cost of antiretroviral medication per HIV positive receiver, c_2 stands for the percentage of HIV positive receivers of free (non-preventive) health care, and MC stands for the cost of (non-preventive) healthcare per HIV positive receiver. All four parameters can be user manipulated.

Deficit, or debt re-payment, $D_{t-1} = B_{t-1}$, if $B_{t-1} < 0$ (*i.e.* deficit at time t exists if in the previous period the budget balance was negative). In the initial period, D equals the budgetary cost of HIV prevention programs, a user-defined parameter.[28] HIV prevention

---

28. There is no explicit constraint on running intertemporal budget deficit. However, a persistent budget deficit is not admissible in the model, and the user is advised then to re-consider parameters open to manipulation (e.g., tax rates, percentage coverage, or costs of preventive programs).

program is aimed at the reduction of the speed of transmission of HIV. Quantitatively, the effectiveness of anti-HIV programs is defined by the user by adjusting one or more of the three transmission parameters, π_1, π_2, and π_3.

Quantitative Analysis of HIV Trends in Central Asia

To better understand the mechanics and dynamics of HIV development in the FSU countries, the study took a closer look at the Russian experience first. On one hand, Russia could serve as a reference point and forecasting device. On the other hand, the Russian experience sheds light upon the general pattern of spread of HIV/AIDS in CA countries.

For a long time, Russia was known as a country of low prevalence of HIV-infection.[29] The regular analysis of data showed that the first group of HIV infected Russian contracted HIV through sexual contacts with African and North Americans in the beginning of 1980s (Pokrovsky 1996). The first case of a HIV positive Russian citizen was diagnosed in 1987. Presumably, in the following two or three years the HIV virus was actively transmitted through sexual contacts and detected in circles close to this original group of HIV-positive Russian(s).

Until mid-1990s, the virus was slowly spreading among heterosexuals and homosexuals alike, with approximately 100–200 new cases registered every year (while approximately 20 million persons were tested annually). In the end of 1995, the first cases were registered where HIV had been contracted by intravenous drug use, and HIV began to spread rapidly, reaching 86,000 by end-2000, and 242,888 by June 1, 2003. According to the Federal AIDS Center, Russia has the highest HIV growth rate in the world, except for Ukraine. 59,257 newly registered HIV-positive persons were found in 2000. In 2001 the number of registered cases was 88,422, twice as much as the total number of cases registered before from 1987. Most recently (end of 2001 onward), heterosexual contacts again took the lead as the main source of infection, and the epidemic increasingly became a nation-wide threat.

Figure 26 shows logs of the number of cumulative registered cases. Following on the discussion above, the study segmented four stages of HIV spread with notably different growth patterns.

Quantitatively, these four stages of HIV development in Russia are distinct, and the distinctions are statistically significant. Table 13 below provides the results of multi-stage regression analysis that quantifies the sequential change in the rate of HIV spread in Russia in 1987–2003. In each stage, the specification of the model is log-linear, with time (T) in

---

29. Surveillance was established in 1987 and includes testing of selected groups (including blood donors, professional soldiers, pregnant women, known intravenous drug users, carriers of sexually transmitted diseases, patients with symptoms similar to HIV/AIDS, male homo/bisexual, prisoners, medical staff in contact with HIV/AIDS patients or HIV-containing materials, being in contact with HIV/AIDS persons, foreigners), mandatory reporting of all tests to HIV antibody and HIV positive cases to the Federal AIDS Center, and interviewing of all HIV positive cases to detect possible risk factors responsible for the transmission of HIV, and reporting of these findings to the Federal AIDS Center.

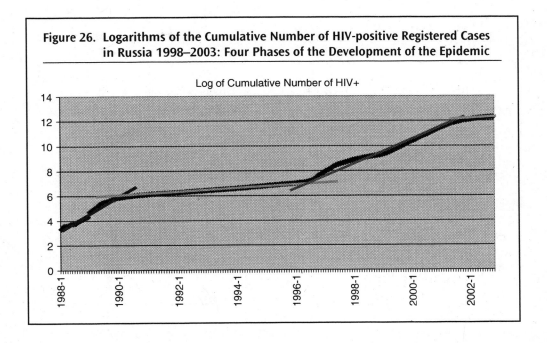

Figure 26. **Logarithms of the Cumulative Number of HIV-positive Registered Cases in Russia 1998–2003: Four Phases of the Development of the Epidemic**

months being an explanatory variable, and the natural logarithm of the cumulative number of registered HIV positive cases (Ln_CUM) being a dependent variable:

$$Ln\_CUM_i^J = \alpha^J + \beta^J + T_i^J + \varepsilon_i^J, \; i = 1, 2, \ldots, I^J, \hspace{2cm} (12)$$

where _ is an error term, and $J = 1, \ldots, 4$ indexes the stage. For each J, the starting and terminal months T_1^J and T_{IJ}^J are chosen to maximize the significance of difference of slopes _^{J}, $J = 1, \ldots, 4$, and $T_{IJ}^J = T_1^{J+1}$. The coefficient _^{J} measures the rate of growth of HIV in the population. Surprisingly, a strong correlation between dependent and explanatory variables (adjusted R^2 close to 1) indicates that the time profile of the development of HIV pandemic in Russia almost perfectly fits the exponential pattern.[30] Therefore, the estimated log-linear trend can be used to make (at least) short-run predictions about the spread of HIV over time.[31]

Similar research using Kazakh, Kyrgyz, and Uzbek data reveals patterns of HIV growth strikingly congruent to what has been observed in Russia, even though in Central Asia the explanatory power of the log-linear model is lower, presumably due to poorer data quality. Nevertheless, all three CA countries lag behind Russia, notably Uzbekistan and the Kyrgyz Republic: so far, they have not reached the stage when heterosexual HIV transmission starts

---

30. In the past, epidemiologists in Russia (notably V. Pokrovsky) attempted to derive a rule of thumb to predict the pace of HIV in Russia: they guessed that the number of HIV positive registered cases doubles every year and a half. The results in Table 13 quantify this expert estimate.

31. There are certain reservations, however. For instance, the break points in log-linear trends may occur when the disease saturates in certain risk groups (*e.g.*, the epidemic has saturated among IDU or CSW, and starts to spread via sexual contacts of IDU partners and CSW clients).

Table 13. OLS Estimates of Four Stages of Development of the HIV Epidemic in Russia: 1987–2003

	Number of cumulative HIV positive registered cases		HIV Development		Regression Statistics	
	Beginning of Period	End of Period	Growth Rate	Doubling[2]	P-value	Adj. R[2]
STAGE 1: May 1987–January 1990	12	354	0.112*	6	0.000	0.99
STAGE 2: January 1990–August 1996	354	1545	0.015*	46	0.000	0.99
STAGE 3: August 1996–July 2001	1545	146830	0.072*	10	0.000	0.98
STAGE 4: July 2001–March 2003[1]	146830	236821	0.023*	30	0.000	0.96
Average, May 1987–March 2003	12	236821	0.046*	15	0.000	0.94

[1]March 2003 is the most recent data available
[2]Time span in months when the number of cumulative registered HIV positive cases doubles
*Significant at 1-percent level

to prevail; also, HIV prevalence in the region is not as high as in Russia (as of May 2003). Therefore, taking Russia as a reference point, it may be concluded that in absence of effective policy measures focused on controlling illicit drug use and prevention of HIV spread from high risk groups (above all IDU) to the rest of population, Central Asia countries are likely to replicate the Russian experience.[32]

In all three Central Asian countries under study, the stage of slow HIV positive growth at monthly rates of 0.01–0.02 was followed in the late 1990s (2001 in the Kyrgyz Republic) by a dramatic acceleration of HIV spread with nearly ten-fold increase in the rates of growth, primarily among IV drug users. So far HIV in Central Asia is transmitted through drug injection. Nevertheless, in the nearest future sexual transmission will likely take the lead and become the main source of infection, and the latter will make increasingly difficult to identify highly vulnerable groups and control the epidemic.

Figure 27 depicts intertemporal changes in the log of cumulative number of registered case in Kazakhstan, Kyrgyz Republic, and Uzbekistan, respectively, and Table 14 summarizes the results of regression analysis.

---

32. As was noted before, even with comparable HIV prevalence rates, countries with dramatically different populations might have dramatically different HIV prevalence. Therefore, the weights assigned to various policy measures should be adjusted accordingly.

Figure 27. Logarithms of the Cumulative Number of HIV-positive Registered Cases in Kazakhstan, Kyrgyz Republic, and Uzbekistan

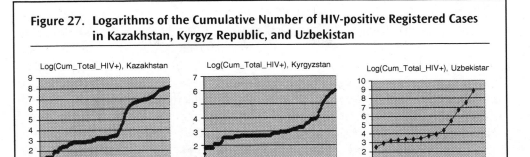

Table 14. OLS Results on Three Stages of Development of the HIV Epidemic

	Number of cumulative HIV positive registered cases		HIV Development		Regression Statistics	
Kazakhstan: 1987–2002	Beginning of Period	End of Period	Growth Rate	Doubling[2]	P-value	Adj. R[2]
STAGE 1: January 1987–June 1996	2	34	0.022	31	0.000	0.87
STAGE 2: June 1996–November 1997	34	499	0.167	4	0.000	0.99
STAGE 3: November 1997–December 2002	499	3257	0.030	23	0.000	0.97
Average, January 1987–December 2002	2	3257	0.039	18	0.000	0.93
Kyrgyz Republic:1987–2003						
STAGE 1: February 1987–February 2001	1	62	0.011	65	0.000	0.87
STAGE 2: February 2001–April 2003	62	403	0.071	10	0.000	0.94
Average, February 1987–April 2003	1	403	0.017	41	0.000	0.77
Uzbekistan: 1987–2002						
STAGE 1: 1987– 1992	0	26	0.032	22	0.069	0.98
STAGE 2: 1992–1999	26	76	0.012	59	0.001	0.83
STAGE 3: 1999–May 2003	76	2209	0.091	8	0.000	1.00
Average, 1987–2003	0	2209	0.034	21	0.000	0.78

Scenarios

The model depicts one baseline forecast and two scenarios. The baseline is the "no-HIV case," which assumes that there is no disease in the population. The scenarios are an "optimistic scenario" and a "pessimistic scenario." Scenarios are not forecasts. Rather, they are benchmarks to vary treatment costs and other economic input parameters, and to contrast the results of user determined scenarios. The results of calibrating the model indicate a set of four parameters to which the economic consequences of HIV react most sensitively: (a) the rate of population growth, (b) the rate of growth of drug users, (c) the HIV transmission rates (among drug users, between drug users and non-drug users, and among non-drug users), and (d) the multiplier used to translate registered into actual HIV positive cases. Congruently, the input parameters that distinguish both scenarios from each other are the following:

- *The rate of population growth* (low rate for the pessimistic case and high rate for the optimistic case). The growth rate brackets are different across countries and vary from [−0.5 percent, −0.1 percent] in Kazakhstan to [0.8 percent,1.2 percent] in Kyrgyz, and to [1.8 percent, 2.4 percent] in Uzbekistan.
- *The rate of growth of drug users*, following the registered numbers officially reported. The model has been calibrated with 5 and 9 percent (7 percent for Russia), respectively for the optimistic and the pessimistic scenario. These numbers are based on the estimates provided by the Federal AIDS Center in Russia and regional statistics. According to official statistics provided by the Kazak Ministry of Justice, in the first half of 2003 the number of drug users in Kazakhstan increased by 3.1 percent.
- *The multiplier* that is used to deduce the number of actually infected individuals from the number of registered HIV positive observations (this number is country specific and depends on the size and composition of tested sample). The model has been calibrated for Kazakhstan with a multiplier of 2 for the optimistic case and 10 for the pessimistic case; for Uzbekistan with a multiplier of 2 for the optimistic case and 7 for the pessimistic case; and for Kyrgyz with a multiplier of 4 for the optimistic case and 6 for the pessimistic case. In Kazakhstan, with more than three-thirds of registered cases being among IDU, UNAIDS estimates that the real number of HIV positive cases is at least twice as high as the number of registered cases, while other experts believe that the real number is at least ten times higher. According to government statistics, there are 47,241 registered IDU, while independent estimates place the real number closer to 250,000. However, in September 2002, the government abolished mandatory testing of inmates in the country penitentiary system, thereby lessening its surveillance basis. In Uzbekistan, according to the information provided by the Uzbek AIDS Center, IDU are strongly prevalent among registered cases of HIV, with a share of 65 percent. According to an assessment conducted by UNODC in 2002, the total number of drug dependant people in Uzbekistan is estimated to be between 65,000–91,000, with only about 19,000 of them officially registered by the drug users service (Narcology Dispensaries). More than half of drug users inject drugs. The estimated total number of drug injectors (both occasional and drug dependant) in the country is about 200,000. Their injecting behavior in terms of sharing syringes and needles, and using human blood for the preparation of drug solutions, is extremely unsafe.

Registered HIV cases are predominant in Tashkent City, Tashkent Province, and Surkhandariya Province with a prevalence of 1,100, 420, and 90 per 1 million population age 15–49, respectively. Sentinel serological surveillance conducted in the city of Tashkent in 2001 revealed a prevalence of HIV among 45.5 percent of IDU. Thus, it is likely that the real number of HIV cases in Uzbekistan is much higher than the registered number. In addition, it has to be taken into account that over 5,000 ELISA-positive blood samples have not yet been confirmed by Western Blot.

■ *The transmission rates of HIV across different groups* of the population. The transmission rate among drug users is 2 for the optimistic case and 5 for the pessimistic case—that is, one intravenous drug user is estimated to infect 2 to 5 other drug users per year. The transmission rate among non-drug users, in line with international estimates, has been set at 0.3 and 0.4, respectively; the rate with which HIV is transmitted from drug users to non-drug users has been kept at this same level. As mentioned before, special emphasis is given to IDUs because this sub-group has the highest HIV prevalence, and comprises high-risk core transmitters of HIV to the rest of population through sexual contacts. Moreover, according to various field studies, an important share of another high-risk core transmitter sub-group (commercial sex workers) inject illicit drugs at least occasionally.

Results and Discussion

Choosing a forecasting period up until 2020, Tables 15, 16, and 17 provide the summary results of the consequences of HIV, under the assumptions specified above and without any prevention.[33]

Without preventive and antiretroviral treatment, the human costs could be dramatic. In the optimistic case, *mortality rates* per month would increase nearly tenfold from 2005 to 2020, accounting for about a hundred deaths a month, and the cumulative number of HIV infected individuals would rise to tens of hundreds by 2020. The pessimistic scenario results in dramatically higher rates, with millions of people infected in Kazakhstan and Uzbekistan by the year 2020.

Under the assumptions discussed above, without preventive policies or treatment, the economic impact on GDP, growth and investment would also be substantial. Even in an optimistic scenario, in all three countries GDP in 2010 would be up to about 1.5 percent lower (from –1.4 percent in the Kyrgyz Republic to –1.75 percent in Kazakhstan). Without intervention, the cumulative loss would rise to roughly 2 percent by 2015 (–1.69 percent in the Kyrgyz Republic, –2.19 percent in Kazakhstan, and –2.7 percent in Uzbekistan). Perhaps more significant for long-term development, the uninhibited spread of HIV would diminish the economy's long term growth rate, slowing it down by 2015 by roughly 3 percent in Kazakhstan and in the Kyrgyz Republic, and by about 5 percent in

---

33. Projections over 15–20 years may be of limited policy value, as the model is based on assumptions that change over time. Among them are the long-term projections of the rate of growth of population, drug users, and GDP. Also, the multiplier that is used to estimate the number of actually infected individuals is estimated with uncertainty, notably in Kazakhstan and Uzbekistan. Regarding the fiscal costs of HIV treatment, the model reckons on current costs of antiretroviral drugs, which are expected to continue decreasing in the future.

Table 15. Economic Costs of HIV in Kazakhstan

Year		2010	2015	2020
Monthly Mortalities	Optimistic	11	45	120
(average)	Pessimistic	54	250	970
Cumulative HIV	Optimistic	0.20	0.40	0.80
(thousands)	Pessimistic	1.70	4.90	11.80
GDP level (2002 = 1)	Baseline	1.71	2.28	2.84
	Optimistic	1.68	2.23	2.75
	Pessimistic	1.64	2.12	2.57
% change (compared to baseline)	Optimistic	−1.75	−2.19	−3.17
	Pessimistic	−4.09	−7.02	−9.51
GDP growth (percent)	Baseline	6.57	5.04	3.79
	optimistic	6.40	4.89	3.66
	pessimistic	6.02	4.51	3.20
% change (compared to baseline)	optimistic	−2.59	−2.98	−3.43
	pessimistic	−8.37	−10.52	−15.57
Investment	optimistic	−0.28	−0.36	−0.65
% change (compared to baseline)	pessimistic	−0.86	−1.06	−1.96
Effective Labor Supply	baseline	0.99	0.99	0.98
(2002 = 1)	optimistic	0.97	0.96	0.95
	pessimistic	0.93	0.90	0.86
% change (compared to baseline)	optimistic	−2.02	−3.03	−3.06
	pessimistic	−6.06	−9.09	−12.24

Uzbekistan, of the growth rate in the baseline "no-HIV case," which assumes that no disease will spread in the population. In the pessimistic case, the average magnitude of annual GDP loss would account up to 1 percent in all three countries, so that *GDP* would be up to about 5 percent lower (from −4.1 in Kazakhstan to −5.6 percent in Uzbekistan) in 2010, and the cumulative loss would rise—without intervention— to roughly 10 percent by 2020 (−8.4 percent in Kyrgyz Republic, −9.5 percent in Kazakhstan, and −11.6 percent in Uzbekistan). Symmetrically, the uninhibited spread of HIV under the pessimistic scenario would slow down the *growth rate* on average (over the forecasting period 2004–2020) by about 11 percent in Kazakhstan and Kyrgyz Republic, and by more than 23 percent in Uzbekistan. In all three countries *investment* would decline (though the magnitude of decline would vary across countries), indicating more of a stumbling block for future growth.

Similarly, the *effective, i.e.* quality adjusted *labor supply* would suffer losses due to HIV as compared to the baseline scenario. The magnitude of losses is comparable across countries and averages from 2 to 6 percent in 2010 and 4 to 13 percent in 2020 in the optimistic and pessimistic cases, respectively. However, the overall decline in Kazakhstan could be due more to a decline in the number of workers associated with negative population

Table 16. Economic Costs of HIV in the Kyrgyz Republic

Year		2010	2015	2020
Monthly Mortalities	optimistic	21	42	72
(average)	pessimistic	47	160	350
Cumulative HIV	optimistic	0.04	0.06	0.10
(thousands)	pessimistic	0.10	0.30	1.10
GDP level (2002 = 1)	baseline	1.43	1.78	2.14
	optimistic	1.41	1.75	2.09
	pessimistic	1.37	1.67	1.96
% change (compared to baseline)	optimistic	−1.40	−1.69	−2.34
	pessimistic	−4.20	−6.18	−8.41
GDP growth (percent)	baseline	4.80	4.07	3.33
	optimistic	4.64	3.93	3.22
	pessimistic	4.28	3.60	2.88
% change (compared to baseline)	optimistic	−3.33	−3.44	−3.30
	pessimistic	−10.83	−11.55	−13.51
Investment	optimistic	−2.00	−2.50	−2.86
% change (compared to baseline)	pessimistic	−8.00	−8.33	−8.57
Effective Labor Supply	baseline	1.09	1.16	1.23
(2002 = 1)	optimistic	1.07	1.12	1.18
	pessimistic	1.03	1.06	1.09
% change (compared to baseline)	optimistic	−1.83	−3.45	−4.07
	pessimistic	−5.50	−8.62	−11.38

growth rate, while in the Kyrgyz Republic and Uzbekistan, the effective labor supply would undoubtedly decline due to the productivity losses associated with those parts of the work force that would be HIV infected.

Table 18 indicates the potential impact of treatment with antiretroviral drugs. The diversion of private and public resources, which otherwise would have been available to finance investment, into treatment, and economically speaking toward consumption, comes at a cost to the economy and this economic cost depends on the price at which antiretroviral treatment is available. The table demonstrates the budgetary impact of antiretroviral treatment. The figures are derived under the assumption that 10 percent of GDP will be spent on expenditures unrelated to HIV, but which are so important that they have to be undertaken under all circumstances.

Based on current costs for antiretroviral drugs of $9,000 per person per year, treatment costs in the pessimistic scenario are not sustainable in all three CA countries. Recently negotiated costs of $3,000 per person per year will hardly be sustainable as well. Therefore, in the medium term, Central Asian countries will either need to negotiate further reductions in the costs of antiretroviral drugs, or take preventive measures to slow down the spread of HIV epidemic to be able to maintain a balanced budget.

Table 17. Economic Costs of HIV in Uzbekistan

Year		2010	2015	2020
Monthly Mortalities	optimistic	3	4	62
(average)	pessimistic	10	21	400
Cumulative HIV	optimistic	0.20	0.50	0.80
(thousands)	pessimistic	1.00	5.00	29.60
GDP level (2002 = 1)	baseline	1.26	1.48	1.72
	optimistic	1.24	1.44	1.67
	pessimistic	1.19	1.35	1.52
%change (compared to baseline)	optimistic	−1.59	−2.70	−2.91
	pessimistic	−5.56	−8.78	−11.63
GDP growth (percent)	baseline	3.22	3.16	3.06
	optimistic	3.04	3.01	2.92
	pessimistic	2.52	2.49	2.28
% change (compared to baseline)	optimistic	−5.59	−4.75	−4.58
	pessimistic	−21.74	−21.20	−25.49
Investment	optimistic	−0.08	−0.65	−0.71
% change (compared to baseline)	pessimistic	−0.78	−1.95	−3.28
Effective Labor Supply	baseline	1.19	1.34	1.51
(2002 = 1)	optimistic	1.16	1.30	1.45
	pessimistic	1.10	1.19	1.28
% change (compared to baseline)	optimistic	−2.52	−2.99	−3.97
	pessimistic	−7.56	−11.19	−15.23

Table 18. Fiscal Costs of Antiretroviral Programs in 2020 (pessimistic scenario)

Annual costs of retrovirals (USD)	w/o	$9,000	$3,000	$300
Kazakhstan				
Budget (% of GDP)	10.79	Deficit	Deficit	9.44
Difference %				−12.51
Kyrgyz Republic				
Budget (% of GDP)	4.03	Deficit	2.35	3.87
Difference %			−41.69	−3.97
Uzbekistan				
Budget (% of GDP)	16.35	Deficit	Deficit	11.62
Difference %				−28.93

This model can be used to mimic different policies and changes in behavior triggered by different policies. By varying one of the most important parameters, the results can be summarized as follows. A change in behavior that would cut all transmission rates by a factor of four (for example, by limiting needle sharing) would improve economic performance in a moderate way by gaining from 1 to 2 percent of GDP by the year 2020. The reason is that drug abuse and its negative effect on productivity (in Kazakhstan combined with population decline and its negative impact on labor supply) would continue unabated while the number of HIV positive individuals declines. However, such a change will dramatically reduce the HIV-related mortalities that will have far-reaching demographic consequences, especially in the context of population decline in Kazakhstan. Furthermore, a softening of the decline in population growth in Kazakhstan can go a long way in compensating partially for the economic consequences of HIV.

Limiting the growth rate of drug users is among the most effective means of avoiding long term repercussions on economic growth and prosperity in the CA countries. The economic scope of this policy is comparable with—not to say exceed—the positive effect of a reduction of HIV transmission rates. This is explained by the fact that increased intravenous drug use not only accelerates the growth of HIV, but has additional negative effects on the aggregate productivity of labor, as the productivity of drug users is considerably below that of non-drug users. Table 19 quantifies the results.

Table 19. Impact of Reduction in the Growth Rate of IDU

Pessimistic Scenario with Growth Rate of IDU Changing			
From 9 to 2 percent	2010	2015	2020
Kazakhstan			
GDP Levels			
with 9%	1.64	2.12	2.57
with 2%	1.66	2.17	2.64
Percentage gain	**1.22**	**2.36**	**2.72**
Kyrgyz Republic			
GDP Levels			
with 9%	1.37	1.67	1.96
with 2%	1.39	1.7	2.01
Percentage gain	**1.46**	**1.80**	**2.55**
Uzbekistan			
GDP Levels			
with 9%	1.19	1.35	1.52
with 2%	1.21	1.38	1.56
Percentage gain	**1.68**	**2.22**	**2.63**

The Strategic and Regulatory Framework for HIV/AIDS Prevention in Central Asia

This section reviews approaches to HIV/AIDS prevention and control that are supported or even implemented through legislative and regulatory policy in Central Asia. These are primarily directed through the public health systems, but they involve multisectoral components as befits a multisectoral health challenge. The study considers funding for these approaches, vis-à-vis existing limited evidence as to costs and cost-effectiveness, and where applicable, best practices from other regions.

The policy environment of all five Central Asia Republics regarding HIV/AIDS prevention reflects the previous history of Soviet approaches to communicable diseases. The moral climate related to HIV within the Central Asia Republics depends greatly on religion, economic disruption, the rule of law, and the influence of health over policing policies. This climate has changed considerably since the beginning of the HIV epidemic, but further policy support for tolerance, human rights protections, and appropriate medical and social support for HIV-related medical conditions is needed.

Drug-related laws seem to shy away from specific criminalization for drug use, while making the possession of small amounts of illegal drugs a crime. This sets the stage for both repression and corruption. It also creates a situation in which injecting drug users (IDUs) are segregated from medical and social support systems, allowing HIV infection to become more and more concentrated until it bridges through sexual networks outside the IDU community. In terms of policy on IDU approaches, it is necessary as a priority widespread adoption of harm reduction approaches. These include non-specialized, decentralized, and more freely available substitution therapy for drug use. For this to occur, legislative change is necessary to liberalize the use of methadone and other substitution drugs, perhaps even including medically administered heroin. Narcology Centers should not be the only places authorized to provide this treatment. Needle exchange needs legalization and accompanying authority for providers to implement without fear for security. This approach is insufficiently described in all of the Strategic Plans reviewed.

Policy approaches to commercial sex work (CSW) suggest a need for decriminalization, both in terms of the definition of laws dealing with prostitution, and enforcement practices. Gender issues are not addressed by the Strategic Plans, and this should be an area of concentration for policy work. Users of commercial sexual services are not prosecuted in general, while CSWs (most at risk for STI and HIV) are marginalized and isolated by police practices.

Policies to support expanded outreach medical treatment for STI, IDUs, and young people may need further attention throughout the region. The specialized, medical approach to HIV/AIDS cannot be the only approach to reaching vulnerable groups; whether through legislation, funding, or expanded NGO support, decentralized and culturally appropriate facilities will need supportive policies in order to prevent HIV spread across bridging populations.

Stigma against vulnerable groups and people living with HIV/AIDS (PLWHA) seems to be overwhelming in Central Asia. Thus, policies protecting human rights, confidentiality, and anonymous voluntary counseling and testing (VCT) need to be specifically addressed. However, even written policies will not change the underlying professional, governmental, and individual set of prejudices that seem to be widespread in the region. It will likely take a very concerted, professional public information campaign to change social norms, against which all programs will be implemented. Although all Strategic Plans call for several different levels of educational activity, it is really not enough to simply provide information. More importantly, the political commitment needs to be backed up by credible social marketing, normalization of vulnerable groups, and realistic human rights protections.

Two of the four countries of Central Asia that have obtained GFATM grants (Kazakhstan and Uzbekistan) have new anti-retroviral drugs treatment (ARV) targets for 2005 or 2007. Although most of the health systems in ECA more or less guarantee treatment for infectious diseases, the costs of ARV have limited the reality of this guarantee to certain target groups (such as in Kazakhstan, with only children and pregnant women covered before the award of the GFATM grant). The key policy gaps related to ARV have to do with specific financing strategies: negotiations for equity pricing, protocols for treatment based on science and international standards, monitoring of drug resistance, and improvement in laboratory support for ARVs are insufficiently addressed in the Strategic Plans.

It appears as though a substantial investment in policy and legislative modernization is needed in each country. All Strategic Plans suggest the need for cross-sectoral collaboration and action. However, in reality, the territoriality of programs and jurisdictions is very difficult to overcome. The credibility and functionality of the National Coordinating bodies in each country will determine the success of the multi-sectoral activities.

In addition to the Global Fund grants, Central Asia has been benefiting from substantial technical and/or financial assistance from UN agencies, bilateral agencies and international NGOs. UNAIDS recognizes the need for harm reductions strategies and legislative reforms. UNICEF stresses the importance of youth vulnerability, as well as the need to attend to children of AIDS victims (an issue marginally addressed in the Strategic Plans). UNODC recognizes the need for improved drug treatment balanced with interdiction approaches, but there really seems to be a lack of commitment to reducing demand for drug use through liberalizing the criminal code. USAID calls for improvements in surveillance, blood safety, and youth-oriented education. Ultimately, the countries will have to decide for themselves how best to change national policy, but the evidence-base provides for substantial support for harm reduction and much more extensive substitution therapy. The evidence is still unclear as to the applicability of decriminalization of drugs as an effective HIV prevention strategy, but it is clear that current legislative approaches do not support effective interventions on IDU-related HIV prevention.

In this study, first we present a brief review of evidence-based strategies to HIV/AIDS prevention and control; many of these strategies have been previously reviewed in detail for the Eastern Europe and Central Asia Region as a whole (Adeyi and others 2003). Those with particular relevance to Central Asia will be highlighted. Next, we discuss key elements of the UNAIDS-published Strategy for this region, including partner activities by the World Bank, Unites States Agency for International Development (USAID), and the Global Fund to Fight AIDS, TB, and Malaria (GFATM). Third, we synthesize material provided by specific country strategic plans for Kazakhstan, Kyrgyz Republic, Tajikistan, Turkmenistan, and Uzbekistan. Fourth, we discuss Central Asian country HIV/AIDS Strategies with regard to gaps based on evidence to identify other possible inputs. In particular, attention is paid to the intravenous drug use problem in Central Asia, as it not only drives the epidemic in this sub-region but also has geopolitical significance.

Strategies to Prevent HIV/AIDS in Central Asia

The key elements characterizing the HIV/AIDS epidemic in Central Asia (CA) are:

- Low HIV prevalence measured by existing reporting systems,
- A rapid rise in new HIV infections,
- Expanding numbers of injecting drug users (IDUs),
- Increased reported sexually transmitted infections (STIs),
- Increased commercial sex work (CSW),
- Increased migration and mobility throughout the region, including drug trafficking, refugees, human trafficking, war traffic, and commercial transport,
- Low levels of awareness of risks, especially among young persons,
- High levels of stigmatization against risk groups and infected persons,
- Inadequate sentinel and population-based surveillance of HIV, risk behavior, and drug use,
- Inadequate health systems response to HIV/AIDS harm reduction, and other preventive and clinical strategies directed to the IDU problem, and
- Relatively low political commitment and low-level civil society involvement.

These determinants have been thoroughly discussed elsewhere (Adeyi and others 2003; Hamers and Downs 2003; Grund 2001). The epidemic, as in other parts of Eastern Europe and Central Asia, is fueled by heterosexual transmission, is at an early stage of development, and depends largely on the bridging from highly vulnerable groups to the general population.

However, the real extent of the epidemic is poorly understood, owing to lack of serologic and behavioral data representative of the highest risk groups (especially IDUs, mobile populations, and CSWs, as well as their needle-sharing and sexual networks). Even though the prevalence of HIV infection in the general population (as well as among highly vulnerable groups) is at present relatively low (highest prevalence is in Ukraine at 1 percent), indications from drug using populations and localized epidemics in Russia, Belarus, and Ukraine suggest that the prevalence within pockets of highly vulnerable groups and vulnerable populations is growing rapidly and is likely to be underestimated due to deficient reporting.[34]

In Central Asia, outbreaks of HIV-related injecting drug use are reported and are cause for concern. Policies to support prevention in low-HIV prevalence countries found in Central Asia are impeded by lack of priority setting, marginalization of vulnerable populations, lack of public knowledge about HIV/AIDS risks, and deterioration of public health systems that need to respond to new infectious disease threats across various sectors (Brown and others 2001; World Bank 2003a).

The Evidence Base for Prevention of HIV/AIDS in Central Asia

Evidence to support effective strategies is largely lacking in the region. However, much can be gleaned from Southeast Asia, Western Europe, Americas and Africa regarding the strategic and regulatory framework for HIV/AIDS prevention in Central Asia. A broad view of effective strategies that may be considered in Central Asia are shown in Box 10. Because the HIV/AIDS epidemic is closely related to the epidemic of intravenous drug use, we must also consider specific interventions directed towards this concomitant epidemic. Box 8 considers specific strategies with respect to the drug-use epidemic.

Political and economic changes in the sub-region have created open borders for drug trafficking, and the HIV epidemic has essentially followed, due to burgeoning demand, the traffic in addictive drugs (OSI 2002). More than 90 per cent of all heroin sold in Europe is sourced to Afghanistan through Central Asia, and the highest rates of documented HIV prevalence among IDUs are along the trafficking routes (Stachaowiak and Beyrer 2002). In areas growing opium poppies, most users smoke or snort the drug; as the opium is converted to diluted heroin along the traffic route, more injection behavior is seen due to its reduced cost per dose compared to smoking or snorting. An estimated 300,000–500,000 of the 55 million persons living in Central Asia are now IDUs (USAID 2003a).

The primary mode of HIV transmission in this region is injection drug use, through needle sharing and unprotected sexual activity. Risk factors also include commercial sex work, social repression of homosexual behavior, and high rates of sexually transmitted diseases, especially syphilis. Thus, the most important strategies related to IDUs are the following:

- harm reduction through needle exchange and substitution therapy;
- drug addiction treatment, detoxification, and counseling;

---

34. CDC (2003b). Rapid increase in HIV rates—Orel Oblast, Russian Federation, 1999–2001. *Morbidity and Mortality Weekly Report* 52(28):656–660; UNAIDS (2001). *HIV Prevention Needs and Successes: a tale of three countries.*

- primary prevention through youth-orientation educational programs;
- changing sexual risk behavior among IDUs through psychosocial interventions;
- social marketing of condoms;
- treatment of STIs among IDUs and their partners; and
- voluntary counseling and testing for HIV for IDUs and their partners (with subsequent referral to treatment for HIV-positives).

Currently, the total number of people living with HIV/AIDS in Central Asia is estimated to be about 90,000, but this number will increase to 1.65 million without effective prevention policies focusing on IDU, sexual and social networks, and young people.[35] Reinforcing this estimate are spot surveys showing a high prevalence of HIV among IDUs, for example, 18 per cent in Kazakhstan (USAID 2003c). For IDUs, targeted policies that address the social, legal, and environmental determinants of the Central Asia HIV epidemic and many of these specific interventions are necessary. The growth of heterosexual HIV epidemics in Central Asia will depend on how well the IDU-based source of HIV is controlled and how well the bridging to other parts of the population is understood (Saidel and others 2003).

IDU-related HIV Prevention. The most effective way of preventing HIV transmission among IDUs is the elimination of drug use. However, most programs are oriented towards harm reduction (Needle and others 1998). Harm reduction is a somewhat controversial approach calling for reducing risks and exposures without abstinence of risk behavior; this usually requires extraordinary political resolve for implementation. However, the evidence supports the use of sterile needles, reduced sharing of needles, cookers, and syringes, and encouraging the use of non-injecting forms of addictive substances as effective preventive measures to reduce HIV transmission (Des Jarlais and Friedman 1994; Des Jarlais 2000; Stachowiak and Beyrer 2002).

In fact, these methods may be more effective in low prevalence epidemics than when seroprevalence reaches 20 percent or more. In New York, the expansion of community-based syringe exchange programs was also associated with large-scale reductions in risk behavior (including needle sharing and risky sexual behavior), and HIV incidence among drug users showed a steady decline during the 1990s (Des Jarlais and others 1996).

In Belarus, a local harm reduction project including needle exchange, public information campaigns, behavioral counseling, legal support, and outreach to high risk groups, proved to be cost-effective in terms of reducing the IDU and non-IDU incidence of new HIV infections (Kumaranayake and others 2003). In Sverdlovsk Oblast, Russia, changes in IDU risk behavior have been observed with needle exchange programs, but the results of this study also highlighted the need for more intensive behavioral, political, and resource support to improve outcomes (Power and Nozhkina 2002). In Nepal, a highly targeted street-based outreach program reported a cost effective approach to needle exchange and sexual practice behavioral change (Soderland and others 1993).

---

35. USAID and Central Asia Republics (CAR) Centers for Disease Control and Prevention (CDC) (2003). Program for Infectious Disease Control.

Box 10. Strategies to Prevent HIV/AIDS Epidemic Growth in Central Asia

---

▩ **Major Public Health Interventions**

1. Screening and insuring safe blood supply;

2. Scaling up voluntary testing and counseling (VCT) among high-risk groups, utilizing outreach through NGOs and government facilities;

3. Contact tracing with VCT for new HIV cases;

4. Training and guidelines for parenteral therapies (nosocomial infection prevention);

5. Harm reduction (HR) including needle exchange among IDUs;

6. Scaling up oral drug substitution therapy to reduce needle use among IDUs;

7. Improved STI treatment and education through outreach among CSW;

8. Improved treatment and referral for STI and HIV by health providers, including syndromic treatment for STIs;

9. School-based and other channel education among youth;

10. Condom social market for persons engaging in unsafe sex;

11. De-stigmatization through professional education for health providers;

12. Improved Knowledge, Attitudes, and Behavior (KAB) through mass media communication among general population.

▩ **Legal Framework Changes in Support of HIV/AIDS Prevention:**

1. Decriminalizing IDU;

2. Decriminalizing CSW;

3. Decriminalizing MSM;

4. Increasing availability of oral drug substitution through primary care providers and other non-specialist facilities;

5. Improving job security, rights, and anti-stigma for HIV/AIDS patients;

6. Regional cooperation and legal enforcement of human trafficking violations;

7. Improving confidentiality with respect to VCT, diagnosis, and surveillance;

8. Prevention: HIV prevention through HR, sero-surveillance, and STI treatment; and social support for released HIV-infected prisoners.

▩ **Resolving Information Gaps**

1. Improving sero-surveillance among high-risk groups to better understand patterns, growth, and true incidence of HIV/AIDS;

2. Improving understanding of behavioral risks among high-risk groups (needle sharing; unsafe sex; and KAB among youth);

3. Improving evaluation of interventions through operational research, in particular HR, VCT targeted to high-risk groups, and STI treatment.

▩ **HIV/AIDS Treatment Issues**

1. STI Treatment: syndromic therapy, surveillance, and drug supply.

2. Opportunistic infection treatment: surveillance, referral guidelines, and drugs.

3. Anti-retroviral treatment: referral, guidelines, and surveillance of resistance; drug supply and cost reduction strategies.

4. Screening for high-risk women and appropriate treatment of HIV-infected pregnant women to prevent maternal-to-child transmission.

6. Social support for AIDS patients: nutrition, home care, transport, support groups.

7. Palliative care: guidelines, pain relief, and hospice care.

Box 10. Strategies to Prevent HIV/AIDS Epidemic Growth in Central Asia (*Continued*)

Communications Strategies

▓ **General Public:**

   1. Basic KAB on risks and unsafe sex practices;

   2. Destigmatization for HIV/AIDS patients, IDU, CSW;

   3. Condom social marketing.

▓ **Policymakers**

   1. Encouraging political commitment—focus on human capital and economics;

   2. Destigmatization;

   3. Realistic approach to IDUs—focusing on treatment and prevention;

   4. Special attention to prison populations.

▓ **High-Risk Groups**

   1. Peer counseling for IDUs, CSWs, migrants;

   2. Soldiers and peacekeeping forces;

   3. Condom social marketing.

In Southeast Europe (Croatia, Romania, and Bulgaria), several needle exchange and behavioral harm reduction programs have been implemented but not sufficiently evaluated; these have usually been supported by the Soros Foundation/Open Society Institute (OSI), and have involved local municipalities and nongovernmental organizations rather than government agencies (Novotny and others 2003). An international analysis reported that HIV prevalence could be reduced by 5.8 percent in cities with needle and syringe projects, compared with a 6 percent increase in HIV incidence in cities without such projects (Hurley and others 1997). Consensus is clear that needle exchange schemes are important, and effective means of reducing HIV transmission (Stimson and others 1998). Services for IDUs should also include voluntary counseling and testing for HIV (VCT), a proved method of changing risk behaviors (Coates 2000). In addition, evidence shows that needle exchange and syringe projects can bridge to social, treatment, and other services necessary to reduce the secondary and tertiary burdens of disease due to HIV as well as reduce risk behavior leading to further transmission (Global HIV Prevention Working Group 2002; Van Empelen and others 2003).

Replacement therapy is another effective measure to prevent HIV infection among drug-using populations. Ideally, all drug users should be referred for treatment including methadone maintenance, and counseling to manage their addiction; in reality, drug treatment programs are still rare, although they are increasing throughout Central Asia. The goal of methadone maintenance therapy is not to achieve total abstinence but rather to minimize the disruptive social effects of drug use and to prevent public health externalities caused by sharing needles and associated unprotected sex. There is overwhelming positive evidence to support expanded use of methadone maintenance as a preventive measure for IDU-based HIV epidemics (Drucker 1995). Usually, methadone treatment and maintenance programs in Eastern Europe and Central Asia are based in Narcology Centers, with inpatient-oriented treatment programs that are sometimes regulated in a rather old-fashioned way. Thus, policies and regulatory frameworks need to be modified to diversify treatment, maintenance, and substitution therapy options as well as needle exchange programs. Other drug substitution initiatives include prescribing and administering injecting drugs, such as heroin, under controlled circumstances. In Netherlands, Australia, and Switzerland, this approach has shown promising results (Drucker 1995).

Clearly, all of these approaches to IDU-related HIV prevention require changes in punitive regimes, including the possibility of decriminalization of drug use and needle possession so that drug users are not so marginalized as to be inaccessible to treatment, support, testing, and counseling. In the Netherlands, cannabis has been legal for nearly thirty years; in Canada, medical marijuana has recently been decriminalized; Switzerland and Portugal have also undertaken liberalization of laws concerning use of illegal drugs. Thus far, there has been little evidence of organized crime or violence associated with the domestic legal trade in cannabis. In the Netherlands, the number of hard drug users has declined steadily, and in addition, treatment facilities based in the public health sector have diversified to address hard drug users (perhaps with policing funds no longer needed to enforce cannabis prohibition; Drucker 1995). There will continue to be psychoactive drug use as long as social disruption, economic pain, and fatalism continue to be present in Central Asia; given that these underlying conditions are not likely to show dramatic change in the short term, more aggressive short term approaches to drug use harm reduction are indicated.

CSW-related HIV Prevention. Harm reduction with respect to commercial sex work is another potential policy area of importance in Central Asia. Economic and political changes in Central Asia over the past decade created significant financial hardships, especially for women. This has led to a dramatic increase in migration as well as either voluntary or involuntary involvement in commercial sex work. Often, there is significant overlap in terms of sexual networks with IDUs. In addition, commercial sex work increases risk for STIs, which also lead to increased risk for HIV. Social and economic conditions (as well as the IDU epidemic) are not likely to dramatically change in the near term; other means of primarily or secondarily preventing HIV spread resulting from the exchange of sex for money are needed. Commercial sex work is characterized by criminalization, ostracism (even when migrant CSWs return home), lack of goods and services, lack of power in sexual relationships, and lack of information about preventing HIV infection. In addition, CSWs fear participating in local medical systems due to the potential of identification by police or forced inpatient treatment for STIs (OSI 2002).

OSI has supported specific program work to reduce HIV risk for CSWs. These programs are characterized by outreach to places where CSW are working, peer education, consulting with local police authorities, and increasing access to medical services. Interventions included in this program are:

- Information and referral, with condom, lubricants, bleach kits, and literature distribution;
- Counseling and education;
- Group counseling and education (including peer education);
- Syringe and needle exchange;
- Legal counseling and advocacy;

▓ Professional or vocational training;

▓ HIV testing, STI testing and treatment, gynecological care, and drug detoxification;

▓ Training of clinical, social service, and advocacy group personnel.

The evidence base for CSW interventions is rather limited, but there are some notable successes and positive projections. Thailand has been studied best of all; with the implementation of a 100 percent condom policy in brothels, incidence declined 80 percent compared with rates prior to program implementation. In addition, targeted prevention efforts raised condom use among sex workers in Abidjan from 20 to 80 percent over six years, with a concomitant reduction in prevalence of nearly two thirds. UNAIDS reports other similar successes among CSW in Papua New Guinea, India, and Bangladesh. In Uganda, generalized condom social marketing, a reduction in the median number of sexual partners, and delayed sexual initiation also contributed to success of CSW-related programs (Global HIV Prevention Working Group 2002). In Africa, peer education projects for CSW cost approximately $5.60 per person educated, with $55 per HIV infection averted (Walker 2003). In India, savings of $56 per case with a targeted behavioral intervention for CSWs are reported. In general, safer sex programs that reduce HIV risk through comprehensive means have greater chance of success than simple abstinence-based programs; social and economic conditions will not be conducive to abstinence when women (and men) are forced to seek income or drugs in exchange for sex in Central Asia.

STI Treatment and HIV Prevention. Unprotected sexual intercourse is a risk factor for both HIV and STI, and ulcerative STIs such as syphilis can promote infection with HIV. Several approaches have been documented as effective to address STI and its interaction with HIV. These include condom social marketing, syndromic treatment (without necessarily using laboratory tests), outreach clinics for CSWs and young people (as youth-friendly services), and voluntary testing and counseling for HIV for those identified as having an STI. The evidence to support more extensive STI surveillance, services, and outreach in Central Asia is substantial. In Asia and Africa, modeling studies among countries with HIV seroprevalence ranging from 4 percent (Tanzania) to 80 percent (Kenya), and a combination of syndromic management of STI and condom social marketing showed costs per HIV infection averted ranged from $9.60 to $259.33 (Walker 2003).

A substantial proportion of STIs are asymptomatic, and thus, for especially vulnerable populations such as CSWs, monthly checkups with adequate minimal laboratory back up should be considered. Barriers with respect to STI services include lack of knowledge of HIV risk and of access points for vulnerable groups; lack of coverage for medical treatment for migrants, CSWs, IDUs, and other groups most at risk for both STI and HIV; lack of access or excessive expense for condoms and other contraceptive barrier methods, viricidal lubricants, and woman-controlled preventives; and lack of consistent programmatic linkage to counseling and testing for HIV as a routine preventive intervention for STI patients.

Educational Programs. In low prevalence countries, behavior change is the most effective method to avert the further spread of HIV. However, too often primary prevention education is left to school-based resources, which may not in fact be properly trained to provide education on sensitive lifestyle issues to vulnerable youth. A large knowledge, attitudes, and practices (KAP) survey of youth and adolescents in Central Asia revealed that young people have little formal reproductive health education (UNFPA 2001). They lack information and assistance from adults, and have little access to modern contraception. The most frequent sources of information for young people were their peers. Thus, policies to strengthen formal reproductive health education, including peer education methods, are needed in this region.

There is substantial evidence that behavioral change programs targeted to sub-populations including sex workers and their clients, IDUs, and men who have sex with men (MSM) can slow or lessen spread of HIV. Indepth research and analysis of risk is necessary to understand how to appropriately target these groups, and thus operational research is necessary to determine the distribution of risk in the local settings in Central Asia. Planning to reach these subpopulations requires their participation as well as building generalized support within governments and across sectors to resolve legislative and other barriers. Mobilizing behavioral expertise, using peer educators and better trained health professionals, is key to success in targeted approaches. Stigma and discrimination are key issues to impact through education of opinion leaders or even gatekeepers (such as brothel owners) who are necessary for implementation of policies such as 100 percent condom use for CSWs (Hanenberg and others 1994; Novotny and others 2003).

Peer education involves training members of the drug-using community. In Australia, sustained behavior changes was noted with respect to improvements in self esteem, harm reduction strategies, and social support with such a program. In Central Asia, with the deterioration of educational facilities, peer education projects need to concentrate on out-of-school youth through non-governmental organizations (Defty 2002). In Ukraine, for example, the Hari Krishna organization has developed outreach activities focusing on youth and drugs. Gatekeepers to the drug using community might also be targeted. Health services can also be made more youth-friendly, but efforts to reduce stigma toward IDUs among the health care providers must be a part of this system approach.

Reducing the number of sex partners, using condoms, delaying sexual initiation, and other focused prevention education actions have been shown to be effective in slowing a well established epidemic in Uganda (USAID and Synergy Project 2002). Nevertheless, focused interventions that use multiple means (STI control, VCT, drug treatment referral, harm reduction) are likely to be the most effective preventive efforts in Central Asia, not simply reliance on behavior change.

Voluntary Testing and Counseling (VCT). Currently in Central Asia, most HIV testing occurs among low-risk persons. With the exception of Kazakhstan, which is establishing sentinel surveillance sites throughout the country, and special studies conducted among high risk groups in other countries, such testing does not provide a clear picture of the progress of HIV epidemics in Central Asia. Instead, as discussed above, targeted surveillance (so-called second generation, or sentinel surveillance is needed (WHO and UNAIDS 2000). This will focus on highest risk groups and provide data for decision making and policy changes specific to the concentrated epidemic situation in Central Asia. VCT can support behavior change necessary to reduce risks stemming from IDU and associated unprotected sexual behavior (Coates 2000; Adeyi and others 2003). Policies and strategies in Central Asian countries must include provision for improvement in data collection, analysis, laboratory support, and reporting of results of such second generation surveillance systems. Without such improvements, policy development is precluded and evaluation of progress is impossible.

Political and Legal System Issues. All five countries have addressed various forms of legal and political reform as they strive toward market economies. In Turkmenistan, political activism is severely curtailed, and Islamic fundamentalism in some countries has been used to justify authoritarian attitudes, especially towards marginalized populations. There are considerable disparities in many of these countries with respect to human rights conventions and legislative implementation to support them. All five countries have passed laws than seek to eliminate discrimination against PLWHA and STI patients, but these are irregularly interpreted. Thus, CSWs, MSMs, and IDUs fear problems with the law, registration (by name) of their HIV status if they are tested, and stigma or loss of confidentiality. In Tajikistan, Turkmenistan, and Uzbekistan, homosexual acts are still criminalized.

AIDS cases are reportable in all five Central Asian Countries. Not all have regulations requiring screening of donated blood products, and some have laws requiring expulsion on the basis of HIV positivity. However, National AIDS committees have been established in all of the Central Asia countries, and it is hoped that a transition to a rights based approach to HIV, IDU, CSW, and MSM will prevail. For more detailed existing policy description, see individual country strategies below.

National AIDS Strategies and Programs

All country strategies aim to prevent the spread of HIV/AIDS from a concentrated epidemic to a generalized epidemic by focusing on:

- At risk groups—IDUs, CSWs, and, for some, men having sex with men;
- Improving awareness and understanding among at-risk and vulnerable groups, such as young people;
- Improving the accessibility to and quality of medical care, and counseling and support for infected patients; and
- Providing the legislative environment that will reduce stigmatization and allow for appropriate protocols to be developed.

To achieve these objectives, attention now needs to be focused on translating leadership on HIV/AIDS into identifying practical steps for implementation; the resources being made available to implement the strategies; and capacity building within the organizations responsible for implementing the strategies.

While there is overall consistency in the approach taken by Central Asian countries in the development of their strategies, there is also variation. This variation tends to focus around the detailed level of objectives with, for example, Kazakhstan's measures being, on the whole, more specific than other countries.

Kazakhstan. The Government of Kazakhstan has recognized the need to intervene to avert the epidemics, has put into place coherent strategies, and secured funds through international donors and the GFATM. However, significant barriers remain to delivering a timely response. including: (i) inadequate staffing levels and training in public health analysis and decisionmaking at all levels; (ii) inadequate salaries at all levels to allow public health officials to adequately perform their public health functions rather than focusing on

---

Box 11. Kazakhstan HIV/AIDS National Program

1. Stabilizing the spread of HIV from IDUs by increasing the proportion of IDU involved in prevention programs.
2. Increasing VCT among IDUs and CSWs.
3. Supporting social and environmental changes for vulnerable groups.
4. Restricting risk groups from donating blood or tissue.
5. Implementing educational programs for youth on safer sex and life without drugs.
6. Providing behavior change education for PLWHA, and providing them with ARV to lower viral load and potential infectivity.
7. Providing social support for PLWHA and also for risk groups.
8. Upgrading the legislative basis for law enforcement practices, civil rights protections, and discrimination against risk groups.
9. Working with risk groups to lower stigma and increase their involvement in solving the problems of HIV transmission.
10. Developing a system of Trust Points for needle replacement, psychosocial support, VCT, and IDU treatment (outside the medical establishments).
11. Supporting outreach to risk groups, mobilizing the community to ensure support for prevention programs for them.
12. Strengthening the work of NGOs in prevention and harm reduction.
13. Supporting peer educational efforts among risk group members.
14. Teacher training for school-based health education, as well as training for military personnel.
15. Condom social marketing and increased availability of prevention supplies to risk groups.
16. Syndromic treatment and expanded access to STI services.
17. Protection of the blood supply.
18. Developing appropriate policies to assure drug supply.
19. Developing infrastructure in epidemiology, IEC, economics, social protection.
20. Monitoring indicators.

---

income generation; (iii) limited understanding of the true dimensions of the threat posed by the likely trajectory of the HIV epidemics; (iv) existing resources still fall considerably short of those necessary to deliver intervention at a scale sufficient to have significant epidemiological impact; (v) innovative approaches to modernizing and rationalizing drug treatment and STI services are being resisted by some powerful professional groups; (vi) laboratory infrastructure for HIV testing is being improved with CDC support, but little is being done to support STI diagnostics or to develop locally grounded protocols for syndromic diagnosis and management; and (vii) harm reduction activity is patchy among highly vulnerable groups.

Kazakhstan published a decree on the National Program on Counteracting the AIDS Epidemic for 2001–2005 in September 2001. HIV testing had been based on compulsory and not anonymous approaches, but recently, legislation has become less draconian (Tokayev 2001). Compulsory testing is now recognized as inefficient and ineffective in monitoring the state of the epidemic. Behavioral risks for IDUs were addressed through pilot programs for substitution therapy, but research found that these were insufficient to dissuade injecting behaviors. The new objectives for HIV program implementation are summarized below.

Clearly, Kazakhstan has described a comprehensive program. With the award of a GFAM grant and USAID investments in surveillance and blood safety, much of this work can be addressed. However, it does appear to be heavily invested in health education-based approaches, and it is very vague as to specific changes needed in policy. Decriminalization of drug use is not addressed, but prostitution is already decriminalized. There is insufficient specificity on improving drug treatment alternatives and increasing funding for substitution therapy. There is significant mention of confidentiality, improved access to VCT and social support through Trust Points, and a very direct approach to destigmatization.

In 2003, the Country Coordination Mechanism (CCM) received a grant in the amount of $6.5 million from the GFATM for HIV prevention among vulnerable population groups and provision of treatment to people living with HIV/AIDS. Major scheduled activities include development of infrastructure for ART; drug procurement; and funding of NGOs delivering prevention work with highly vulnerable groups (20 percent of the budget). However some difficulties have been reported in relation to its implementation. These included (i) blockage of the implementation of the proposed syndromic management protocols for STIs by the dermato-venereal establishment; and (ii) blockage of introduction of methadone substitution treatment by the narcological establishment.

In addition, it was reported that there is severe fragmentation of the NGOs working in the field, and an urgent need for support work to develop the capacity of NGOs, promote consolidation and unified methods, and strategic leadership. The AIDS center works closely with NGOs, which are financed by the GFATM grant and other donor assistance. Operations of most NGOs depend on external funding. Termination of funding and/or lack of administrative support may result in collapse of some NGOs.

The Kyrgyz Republic. The Government of the Kyrgyz Republic has grasped early the significance of the epidemics of HIV and sexually transmitted diseases for the country, and therefore Government ownership is strong. The Strategic Plan to control HIV/AIDS epidemic in the country was developed through a broad Government and NGO consultation process; and several Ministries have developed sectoral plans. This process was engineered by the Republican AIDS Center, also with technical and financial support from UNAIDS and other UN agencies. Most NGOs specializing on work with CSWs, IDUs, MsM and other highly vulnerable groups, contributed to the development of this strategy along with public institutions. The Kyrgyz Republic was among the first to develop, not only the Strategic Plan, but also sectoral programs based on the national strategy. The central Government commitment to fight HIV/AIDS is in place, but further advocacy is necessary to engage the Presidential Administration and national Government in the control of the epidemic. The GoK has already established coordinating bodies to guide the implementation of sectoral strategic plans to fight HIV/AIDS, TB and Malaria. The Second State program on the prevention of AIDS and infections of sexual and injecting transmission: 2001–2005, is designed to deliver a comprehensive and coherent package of policies and interventions through intersectoral action.

Box 12. Kazakhstan GFATM grant

---

1. **Reducing the vulnerability and risk behaviors of IDU, CSW and MSM**
   a. Information, education, and counseling
   b. Needle exchange and disinfectants
   c. Substitution therapy
   d. Condom distribution
   e. More supportive legal and social environment
   f. Implemented through Regional AIDS centers, narcology centers, and a few nongovernmental organizations.

2. **HIV/AIDS prevention interventions among youth**
   a. Behavioral education
   b. Students and out-of-school youth
   c. Peer education
   d. Multiple outlets (primary through vocational schools, youth organizations)

3. **Proposed policy changes (through advocacy and training)**
   a. Softening criminal prosecution for illegal procurement and storage of drugs.
   b. Allowing substitution therapy for the management of opium/heroin addiction (now this is prohibited).
   c. Prostitution is now fully decriminalized; however police still harass and arrest CSW, and interventions with police are planned.
   d. More supportive and positive articles in the mass media, including when politicians are interviewed on this subject.

4. **Training of health professionals in behavior change and improved infectious disease control**

5. **Improve the accessibility and acceptability of STI treatment.**
   a. One stop shopping for reproductive health, HIV testing and counseling, and STI treatment.
   b. Youth friendly services encouraged

6. **Strengthening analytic capacity of government health system to better monitor indicators of success**

7. **Improve support for PLWH**
   a. Expand ARV and opportunistic infection treatment using standard protocols and improved laboratory monitoring
   b. Correct antiquated approaches to compulsory HIV testing, deportation of HIV-positives, imprisonment of HIV-positives
   c. Public information campaign to eliminate stigmatization.

8. **Prisons system project to assure HIV/TB treatment interaction**
   a. IEC for prisoners on risks of interaction of these two diseases
   b. No needles, but disinfectant supplies and condom distribution allowed
   c. STI treatment provided
   d. Improved equipment and supplies needed to prevent nonsocomial spread in prison medical facilities.
   e. Sentinel surveillance studies

The Strategic Plan covers a number of important areas of policy reform; however, it does not address sufficiently the area of medications and treatment for ARV and opportunistic infections. Human rights issues are not highlighted, and it does appear as though there are substantial problems, not with the letter of the law, but with the enforcement practices related to IDU and CSW. Thus, although educational approaches are enumerated, the greatest challenge to policy effectiveness is likely to be in changing enforcement agency practices and public opinion. It is curious to see the establishment of a special "militia" related to CSW interventions; perhaps this is simply a translation problem, but it does appear as though decriminalization of prostitution is not planned. The new Plan builds on lessons learned from 1997–2000, when measures of compulsory testing and marginalization of vulnerable groups were more or less official practices.

The Kyrgyz Government recognizes the nascent epidemic, "impetuous drug abuse growth," and social disruption as determinants. Major barriers include insufficient financing, lack of effective education, lack of targeted prevention, weak NGOs, stigmatization, and inappropriate legal structures and discrepant enforcement practices. Targeted interventions began in 1998, and HIV screening moved from universal to focused testing. The new Strategic Plan focuses on youth, IDU, and CSWs. It specifically mentions necessary improvements in the legislative environment, especially the repressive enforcement practices, and improvements in transparency of the response to HIV/AIDS. Blood safety is addressed, including laboratory capacity and personnel training. For youth, measures include behavioral research, school-based education, condom social marketing, teacher training, youth friendly medical services, and mass communication. IDU approaches include behavioral change, peer education, condom distribution, needle exchange, trust points, substitution treatment and rehabilitation program development, and legal protection for IDUs. The CSW objectives include peer education, condom marketing, legal reform, "establishing a specialized militia to assure law and order," establishing a CSW hot line, establishing legal support for CSWs, and training of enforcement agencies.

There is a strong reliance on public education and broad based approach to information dissemination, along with special attention to the educational needs of vulnerable groups. STI treatment, sentinel surveillance, CSW outreach, and trust points for clinical services are called for. Special attention is given to counseling and where indicated, testing of pregnant women for HIV. Finally, psychosocial assistance for PLWHA is addressed, but not mentioning ARV treatment.

The Government in association with NGOs submitted a well designed proposal to the GFATM: $5 million has been awarded to support the first 2 years of the program, with high levels of support going to NGOs. Targets are ambitious, including 60 percent drugs harm reduction coverage; and 80 percent of demand for methadone substitution to be met by 2007. The grant areas of work include (with indication of percent of budget allocation): (i) strengthening of political and legal support (2 percent); (ii) reducing vulnerability of young people (20 percent); injecting drug users (36 percent); sex workers and their clients (6 percent); prison inmates (4 percent); MSM (12 percent); (iii) ensuring safety of donors' blood (18 percent); and (iv) medical and social support to HIV positive persons (18 percent). However, NGOs complain that no monies have been disbursed to support their work and that this is putting them into a serious funding crisis.

The CCM that was established to apply for the GFATM grant is chaired by the Deputy Prime Minister, and brings together members of the existing collective coordinating bodies:

Box 13. Kyrgyz Republic GFATM Grant

1. Improve multisectoral approach, including changing legal framework to support HIV programs.
2. Compulsory youth educational programs, youth friendly health services, peer education, and increased condom availability for sexually active youth.
3. Compulsory education for military servicemen.
4. IDUs
   a. Needle exchange programs
   b. Methadone maintenance programs
   c. Confidential testing and counseling for HIV
   d. Sexual behavior change and condom marketing.
   e. Improved clinical service availability for IDUs
2. Reducing vulnerability of CSWs and clients
   a. NGO based clinical service provision
   b. Condom access improvement
   c. STI treatment improvement and monitoring
   d. Peer education
3. Reduce prisoner vulnerability
   a. IEC
   b. Harm reduction (methadone, disinfection, needle exchange
   c. STI treatment improvement
4. Reducing vulnerability of MSM
   a. Preventive medical care
   b. Condom marketing
   c. IEC
   d. Research on behavior, prevention, etc.
5. Ensuring blood safety
   a. Voluntary blood donor program
   b. Improved, universal screening of donated blood
   c. Monitoring and information system
6. Provision of medical support to PLWHA
   a. VCT
   b. Sentinel surveillance and sociological surveys
   c. NGO strengthening
   d. 100 per cent coverage with ARV for those who need it.
   e. Targeting pregnant women who are at risk for HIV.
   f. Psychological counseling

National Multisectoral Coordinating Committee on Prevention of HIV/AIDS, STI and Infections Transmitted by Injections; National Coordinating Committee on TB Control under the Presidential Administration; National Emergency Epidemics Control Commission, as well as members of technical expert groups, NGOs and international partner organizations. Implementation commenced in August 2003.

However, the functionality and effectiveness of the CCM are questioned by national and international stakeholders; and the mechanisms to secure the release of funds to NGOs are lacking. This may be due to weak institutional capacity. The donor community and most NGOs suggest that the CCM requires immediate assistance to become functional and be able to coordinate the multi-sectoral response in these critical areas. These organizations propose the establishment of a CCM Secretariat with well-trained staff to ensure adequate functioning of the CCM. Presently, secretarial functions are assumed by the Republican AIDS Center for the HIV/AIDS Program and by the TB Institute for TB Program. However, both institutions have not yet been able to provide adequate secretarial services, and after receiving the GFATM grants, became unwilling to share information on project activities and funding allocations. This upsets a broad range of national and international stakeholders that are involved in HIV/AIDS epidemic control; it triggers strong opposition, disrupts the necessary collaborative spirit and may become detrimental to the national response. Timely mitigation of the situation seems to be required to move the process back into a collaborative effort. The means to achieve this could be donor financing and support for an independent Secretariat for TB and HIV/AIDS under the Deputy-Prime Minister.

Tajikistan. The Tajik policy environment currently appears to be changing through a mix of the GFATM and Strategic Plan actions. The National Program on Prevention and Control of HIV/AIDS until 2007 establishes the National Coordination Committee, and defines financing, multisectoral commitments, and program directions (Rahmonov 2000). The Strategic Plan is well written and conceived on a scientific and culturally appropriate basis. It spells out specific multisectoral responsibilities and recognizes the deficiencies in the legislative/policy environment that need correction.

In 1997, the Government adopted a National Program on HIV/AIDS and STIs Control for the period of 1997–1998; and on 30 December 2000, the Government approved the new version of the National Program for the period up to 2007. Tajikistan's National Coordination Committee on HIV/AIDS and STD Prevention is led by the Deputy Prime Minister and the importance of protecting IDUs from HIV infection is accepted at the highest levels, including the Ministry of Justice and Internal Affairs of Tajikistan. However laws criminalizing people who knowingly spread HIV or sexually transmitted infections (STIs), as well as individuals who avoid examination or otherwise attempt to conceal their infection, remain on the books; and, together with police harassment and possible arrest for possession of even a used syringe, drive drug users underground. Actual responses through implementation of interventions have however been rather uncoordinated, and influenced by donor agendas, and coverage remains low.

Tajikistan is a Muslim country, but HIV/AIDS is acknowledged on a political level nonetheless. In this context, there is specific mention that condoms should be used to prevent STI and not as a family planning measure. With respect to HIV, mass screening was previously applied, but the laws now are more consistent with international standards of responsibility by the government for prevention and treatment. The criminal code addresses deliberate spread (that is, with knowledge of infectivity status) of STIs, and this may create additional stigmatization of HIV infected individuals. Administrative and not criminal statutes address prostitution, but in reality, there appears to be extreme prejudice against CSWs. Narcotic use is illegal, and there is insufficient attention to drug sellers in the criminal code. In fact, even a contaminated syringe will be ground for arrest; thus, needle exchange programs could present a significant risk for both participants and providers. There is a poor supply chain for condoms, and need for improved manufacturing capabilities.

The Strategic Plan of the National Response to the HIV/AIDS epidemics for the period of 2002–2004 was elaborated. Specific attention was addressed to preventive activities among vulnerable groups: intravenous drug users, commercial sex workers, refugees, migrants, military servicemen, and youth as well as on provision for blood safety and prevention of parental HIV transmission. The GFATM grant provides for IDU and CSW interventions, VCT, laboratory strengthening to assure blood safety, and development of multisectoral support.

It is noteworthy that the Strategic Plan has specific recommendations regarding the management of sexually transmitted infections:

> The health reform, which is being prepared for implementation in the country, determines a decentralization of the STD service with a partial devolving of functions on treatment and surveillance over STD patients to common physicians working in the public health service network. An extension of anonymous and free of charge medical services to the population is being planned as well as a wider syndrome approach to the STD patients' treatment. Establishment of new clinics for vulnerable groups is also envisaged. However the process of reforming is only being discussed while the existing STD service does not meet requirements of the population.

Donor support to Tajikistan to fight the HIV/AIDS epidemic has been increasing. UNAIDS has been providing assistance to the Government to develop the Strategic Plan, and adequate policies and legislation for HIV/AIDS prevention. Tajikistan was awarded $1.5 million by the GFATM to support implementation of the National Strategic Plan for two years, starting March 2003. The GFATM funding provides inputs to: (i) upgrade lab capacity with new equipment and supplies (test kits); (ii) carry out outreach work with IDUs and CSWs; (iii) carry out IEC for youth in general; and (iv) assure a safe blood supply in the country. However, the UN-TG has initiated additional resource mobilization, as total funding available is not sufficient.

However, the magnitude of the threat, funding available for critical activities such as harm reduction, and loose coordination impair carrying out an adequate response to the growing epidemic. The donor-driven agenda resulted in clustered interventions, which mainly serve the donors' agendas and marginally contribute to strengthening the national response. Competition emerges between national institutions and national NGOs for the limited donor funds, further disrupting the national response to HIV/AIDS and adequate coordination among various agencies involved. Immediate attention from the GoT and donors is therefore required. While donor assistance is forthcoming and expected to increase in coming years, HIV/AIDS has not been well understood by politicians at national and subnational level, requiring the GoT to clearly communicate the importance of the issue.

Box 14. Tajikistan GFATM Grant

1. **IDU interventions:**
   a. IEC
   b. Needle exchange, disinfectants, condom distribution
   c. STI treatment
2. **CSW interventions:** IEC, VCT, STI treatment, decreased vulnerability
3. **Educational actions**
   a. Directed towards youth, including "derelict" children
   b. Teacher training
   c. STI, drug abuse prevention, HIV/AIDS prevention
   d. Health professionals
   e. Mass media
4. **Developing a more positive social environment (destigmatization)**
   NGO development; establishment of trust points to assist in needle exchange, VCT, etc.
5. Laboratory investment to assure a **safe blood supply.**
6. **Behavioral Surveillance**, especially among youth.
7. **VCT** (purchase of test kits).
8. **Cross sectoral support** from law enforcement, NGOs, health professionals, education, mass media, and government officials.

Turkmenistan. A Strategic Plan is not available at this time, although it may be under preparation. The law on HIV/AIDS Prevention was reviewed (Turkmenbashi 2001). It expressly deals with the rights of citizens and foreigners to confidential and anonymous testing for HIV. However, in other parts of the law, there is specific reference to mandatory testing, even of diplomats, for HIV. In addition, while there is mention of protection of job status for HIV infected persons, there is also specific mention of forcing job changes if there is a perceived threat of HIV spread from infected health system employees. Attention to the blood supply, safety of medications, and social support for HIV infected people are mentioned. Financing of preventive measures is addressed as is assurance of free medications for AIDS outpatients.

Reporting of HIV status appears to be mandatory. The Turkmen policy environment appears to be a mix of persistent Soviet approaches to mandatory testing, particularly of migrants and foreigners, while at least mentioning the right to confidentiality, medical treatment, and preventive measures. It seems as though the Law described above has been drafted to sustain both the previous approach to testing and personal responsibility for infectivity as well as newer concepts of human rights and government responsibility.

Uzbekistan. Given a very well written Strategic Plan, intensive donor assistance, and the GFATM grant that was awarded to Uzbekistan in 2004, the policy environment is likely to change considerably (Uzbekistan 2002). The clear focus of the Plan is supported by detailed activities that if implemented and permitted through legislative reform, would have a significant positive effect on the concentrated epidemic. It does appear that there is significant official and public resistance to modern policy approaches, as there appears to

---

Box 15. Uzbekistan Strategic Plan

---

1. Integration of HIV/AIDS into development programs
2. Reforming legislation to increase attention to vulnerable groups for prevention
3. Reducing susceptibility of high risk groups to risk behavior
4. Implementing educational and awareness programs.
5. Increasing accessibility, and quality of health services related to HIV/AIDS (includes blood safety and condom regulations, 100 percent ARV availability)
6. Establishing a national coordinating mechanism.

---

be an entrenched culture of exclusion, misinformation, and criminalization of vulnerable groups. This will be perhaps the biggest challenge for the National Coordinating Committee—changing the social normative environment on HIV/AIDS.

The Strategic Plan recognizes the focus for HIV prevention on IDU, CSW, prisoners, and young people. Formally, drug use is not criminal, but in reality, IDUs are treated as criminals because of purchase and possession of illegal drugs. There does not appear to be ready access to replacement therapy, but arrested drug users are forced into compulsory treatment (essentially, withdrawal therapy), which has been found to be ineffective and encourages isolation of drug users from medical, social, and legal systems. The quantity of drugs considered illegal is less than the usual dose for an addicted user. CSWs are also prosecuted under the administrative code, and homosexual acts are illegal. Thus, the legal code does not support a preventive environment for the most vulnerable groups.

HIV-infected persons are segregated in health care and in prisons. Reporting of HIV status is mandatory, and infected persons are subject to extreme control. Mandatory testing is also supported for certain groups, and thus testing is associated with extraordinary social and legal burdens. As for education, surveys show inadequacy of knowledge among young persons, and NGOs conduct most peer education programs. STI treatment is insufficient, centralized, inpatient oriented, and lacking in availability for the most vulnerable groups. ARV therapy is in general unavailable.

The response thus far to the HIV epidemic has been plagued by the previous Soviet system, insufficient governance, weakness of multisectoral coordination, lack of human rights-based approaches, and insufficient care and treatment. Prevention is insufficient as are social support mechanisms. A specific project on prisons has been developed, focusing on changing risk behavior through education, involvement of risk groups, and media communications. It is not clear that any harm reduction or improved therapy is involved in this proposed project.

However, the Government of Uzbekistan has been steadily building its commitment and capacity to respond to HIV/AIDS. Most recently, the government developed and approved the Strategic Program on Counteracting the HIV/AIDS Epidemic in the Republic of Uzbekistan for 2003–2006. This document outlines the various roles and responsibilities of the Ministries of Health, Finance, Interior Affairs, Education, Justice and Labor & Social Protection of Population in managing the country's response to HIV/AIDS. Issues related to HIV/AIDS are also incorporated into the Program for Reforming the System of Health

Care in the Republic of Uzbekistan, which was adopted by the Decree of the President of Uzbekistan on November 10, 1998. In 1999, the Parliament passed a law to protect people living with HIV/AIDS from discrimination; the right to equal access to education, employment and social protection is guaranteed by this legislation, as is the right to free care from government health organizations. The Republican Emergency Anti-Epidemic Commission for HIV/AIDS has provided the foundation for the new multisectoral CCM. Uzbekistan has a general information, education and communications (IEC) strategy on HIV/AIDS, which includes specific initiatives for vulnerable groups most at-risk of contracting HIV. A letter on accelerated access to anti-retroviral drugs was signed by the Minister of Health and sent to WHO and UNAIDS.

In 1999, the Parliament passed a law to protect people living with HIV/AIDS from discrimination; the right to equal access to education, employment and social protection is guaranteed by this legislation, as is the right to free care from government health providers. However, legislative reforms required for adequate implementation of strategic program are far from being complete. Significant issues related to the drug use, CSW and MSM are still not addressed. e.g., every year approximately 7,000 IDUs are incarcerated due to the drug use. Issues related to HIV/AIDS were also incorporated into the Program for Reforming the Health Care System in the Republic of Uzbekistan, adopted by Presidential Decree; and are reflected in the Uzbek Health II Project.

However, there are also a number of negative factors within the risk environment. The Republican Emergency Anti-Epidemic Commission for HIV/AIDS has provided foundation for the new multi-sectoral CCM established prior to GFATM application submission. However, the CCM exists on paper but its effectiveness is questionable. State structures concerned with the prevention and treatment of infectious disease play a role akin to policing infected individuals; and notably within the Dermatovenereology service, militia are still involved in capturing segments of the population (particularly CSW) and bringing these compulsorily into to the DVS. There is an attitude of closure and secrecy in relation to availability of official statistics describing HIV/STI and risk behaviors. The NGO sector exists; but is not flourishing or energetic in the same way as that in Kyrgyz. The Government has responded to the need for harm reduction projects by issuing a decree to set up a large number of "trust points" which should deliver VCT as well as advice and harm reduction commodities; and does not significantly support NGOs in this work. These factors will need to be addressed if an effective scaled-up response is to be achieved. In addition low levels of knowledge on HIV/AIDS are likely to be an impediment to prevention.

The Government applied to GFATM for financial support to implement National Strategic plan and received $5,2 million for two years starting May 2004 (the contract has not yet been signed). The overall goal of the program is to prevent the spread of HIV/AIDS into the general population by reducing its impact on the most vulnerable populations. Objectives are: a) effective prevention programs focused on the needs of vulnerable populations; b) access to care, support and treatment for people living with HIV/AIDS; and c) creation of an enabling environment that supports work with vulnerable populations. Activities for the first objective—effective prevention programs focused on the needs of vulnerable populations—include: harm reduction initiatives for IDUs (needle exchange, condom distribution, IEC campaigns and substitution treatment), outreach and peer education programs with sex workers and MSMs, IEC and condom distribution programs in prisons, school and community-based IEC/BCC programs for young people and improvements in STI services. Activities for the second objective—access to treatment for people living with HIV/AIDS—include: broad-based care and treatment services (ARVs, treatment for opportunistic infection, psycho-social support and palliative care) and MCTC. Activities for the third objective—development and implementation of policies to ensure that the enabling environment required to work with vulnerable populations exists in the country—include: education and advocacy campaigns targeting policymakers and opinion leaders in Uzbekistan, training for journalists on HIV/AIDS and improvements in surveillance policy and practice. About 60 percent of the funds are earmarked for Government structures and 35 percent for NGOs.

Regional Agreements and Partnership Programs

Experience with regional cooperation in Central Asia is rather limited and somewhat disappointing (a summary of regional Agreements signed by the Central Asia Governments is attached). However, Central Asia Governments have already initiated regional activities to tackle the drug problem that is at the root of the HIV/AIDS epidemic in ECA. In 2002, they met in Tashkent to agree on a drug supply and drug demand-reduction strategy. As mentioned before, most regional Governments have taken early action to prevent and treat HIV/AIDS by approving appropriate strategies, initiating HIV/AIDS programs based on work with groups at risk (establishment of Trust Points), and securing additional funding from the Global Fund and other sources. In addition, several partner organizations have been actively engaged in advocacy and support to the implementation of the strategies.

After the September 11, 2001, terrorist attacks in the United States, Central Asia became more geopolitically important, and hence the need for political and economic stability has attracted significant international assistance in several different sectors, including military cooperation, humanitarian aid, economic development programs, agriculture, education, and health (USAID 2003a). The World Bank has made significant investments in health systems development projects and in specific public health projects in this region. Various bilateral donors have made and are considering investments through technical assistance, grants and credits geared towards drug use demand reduction, infectious disease prevention and control (especially sexually transmitted diseases and tuberculosis), and HIV. What is important to recognize here is the need for a broad-based approach that considers structural and environmental approaches (including legislation and policy) at several levels:[36]

- Superstructural, including gender and social inequalities that increase risk for women and other vulnerable groups;
- Structural, including laws or policies at both national and institutional levels that interfere with prevention activities;
- Environmental, including local factors that include lack of access to condoms, lack of status for migrants, or adverse social norms regarding ethnic minorities;
- Individual, including lack of knowledge about risks and lack of access to appropriate services.

---

36. UNAIDS Best Practice Collection (2002).

Significant support has become available for prevention and treatment of HIV/AIDS in Central Asia. Governments and partner organizations have been providing significant technical and financial assistance. However, there are significant gaps in coverage of highly vulnerable and vulnerable groups. These gaps are partly due to insufficiency of funding, partly to lack of coordination among the different stakeholders and lack of capacity to implement the agreed strategies.

Regional Drug Control. Interdiction has been one of the more controversial areas in drug control policy. It is difficult to evaluate whether support for such programs creates honest, efficient law enforcement or only empowers officials involved in trafficking to smuggle better (Lubin and others 2002). Certainly the war in Afghanistan opened borders to increased trafficking because of economic pressures and lack of governance. The economy of this country may have more to do with solving the trafficking problem than any law enforcement or public health program. Supply reduction cannot work without a concurrent reduction in demand. With respect to interdiction, a balanced, even-handed political approach is needed. Drug trafficking is ultimately a development issue and thus cannot be addressed by law enforcement alone. It is also closely related to human rights, gender issues, and government corruption. Supply-side programs require greater transparency, coordination, local involvement, long-term funding, and clear linkage to harm reduction and the treatment of drug addiction.

In 1996, Governments of Central Asia signed a Drug Control Agreement, and since 2002 have been carrying out regular assessments through the national Drug Agencies with assistance from UNODC. These national and international agencies have been recently shifting from simple control of drug supply to drug demand reduction (DDR) strategies and prevention of HIV/AIDS. UNODC activities focus on DDR and HIV prevention; border control, law enforcement and strengthening the judicial system. A particular focus is on legal assistance programs and harmonization of legislation.

UNAIDS and the UNODC sponsored a needs assessment on drug abuse in Central Asia (Kumpl and Franke 2002). The main findings and recommendations of this study reinforced the background information on socioeconomic disruption, increases in drug trafficking, and difficulties in measuring the exact size of the drug abuse problem. It called for a balance of activities between supply reduction through the legal system and law enforcement systems; and demand reduction through expanded services for drug users and increased prevention work among young people. The political response has shifted somewhat from neglect and punishment to mobilization for prevention. It was noted that governments in the region have demonstrated a willingness to act on drug use as a critical part of HIV prevention.

Kazakhstan has a nationwide network of governmental rehabilitation centers and a research center. The Kyrgyz Republic is the first country to have implemented methadone substitution projects in a decentralized design. The Tajik Drug Control Agency acts as a focal point for supply as well as demand reduction. Turkmenistan has a centralized system of drug abuse control, but most services are provided by NGOs, targeting special populations and prisoners. Uzbekistan has a national system of governmental and NGO Trust Points that serve IDUs with outreach and peer education. In general, there is still authoritarian command, with fear and punishment as hallmarks for "prevention" activities. Counternarcotics efforts often facilitate human rights abuses for marginalized populations.

There is also over reliance on the medical approach that depends on facilities and treatments at the expense of outreach prevention and harm reduction. Again, harm reduction, increased substitution therapy, decentralization, improved access to services, destigmatization, and increased education of health providers are key to addressing this co-epidemic for HIV/AIDS.

UNODC currently has three projects under the umbrella of drug demand reduction (DDR):

▨ Diversification of prevention, with a budget of $500,000 for the 5 regional countries (of which $50,000 are grants for each country, and the rest finances regional activities and staff). UNODC works with service delivery institutions and aims at strengthening coverage through needle exchange, drug replacement programs and outreach/community activities, and improvement of quality of services. Pilot regions have been selected in the Kyrgyz Republic (Bishkek and Osh); Tajikistan (Khojand and Dushanbe); Kazakhstan (Shymkent and Pavlodar); and Uzbekistan (Tashkent). In these regions, mapping of services, and a training needs assessment is done, and local implementing agencies have been selected (in Tashkent: Narcology Centre);

▨ Drug prevention, with a budget of $400,000 for 2004–2005 to finance information campaigns to raise public awareness, and work with NGOs;

▨ Policy advice on DDR to Governments, with a budget of $400,000 for 2004-2005. Under this component it is planned to have a long-term HIV/DDR adviser partly funded by UNAIDS, to be based in the Tashkent office from June/July 2004. Activities comprise raising awareness on prevention and DDR issues of governments that currently concentrate on law enforcement.

Another project is planned to train professionals in DDR, with an estimated cost of $1.5 million, but funding has not yet been assured. Activities would comprise the development of training courses and integration of focused training into existing curricula. In addition, the UNODC Research Analysis Unit in Tashkent maintains a regional database on main trafficking routes, drug abuse, and HIV/AIDS. The data is collected from local counterparts and law enforcement agencies regularly. UNODC is willing to share this information, including in the context of the pilot partnership that has been developing with the Bank in the region. DFID and the Bank will carry out a regional mapping exercise that will include information on movement of people (CSWs, trafficked people, refugees, labor migrants, traders, truck drivers, travel, customs and law enforcement staff, etc) and goods (especially drugs) along regional corridors—possibly the Northern Corridor and the Silk Route—and STIs and HIV/AIDS cases. Both agencies (DCA and UNODC) have expressed willingness to assist the development of this regional mapping exercise.

UNAIDS Regional Strategy. UNAIDS has developed strategic priorities to control the concentrated and nascent epidemics of HIV/AIDS in Central Asia. In the context of this regional strategy, UNAIDS has been providing support to all countries in Central Asia to approve and implement National Strategic Plans and sectoral strategies, as well as updating the legal framework for prevention of HIV/AIDS. Other UN agencies, such as UNICEF and UNFPA, also have regional programs, but the scope of their HIV/AIDS activities is limited.

UNAIDS Regional Strategy has three main objectives:

- To expand coverage of HIV prevention among injecting drug users to a minimum level of 60 percent;
- To strengthen prevention and care of sexually transmitted infections;
- To develop comprehensive programs for young people's health, development and protection.

In accordance with these directions, UNAIDS established the Task Force on IDU hosted by UNAIDS in Vienna; the Interagency Group for Young People's Health Development and Protection, hosted by UNICEF in Geneva; and the STI Task Force hosted by WHO in Copenhagen. These task forces involve numerous multilateral organizations, bilateral partners, non-governmental organizations, private foundations, academic institutions, and professional associations. The UNAIDS Task Force on HIV Prevention Among Injecting Drug Users In Eastern Europe and the Newly Independent States advocates a comprehensive approach to HIV prevention among IDUs involving:

- Information and awareness raising
- Skills building
- Outreach activities
- Peer education and peer support
- Needle exchange
- Condom promotion and counseling
- Effective drug treatment, including substitution therapy.

These approaches are recognized as effective in other regions and should be adapted to the cultural, social, and economic realities of Central Asia. The underlying concept is to influence IDUs to change behavior, both needle sharing and sexual, to reduce the spread of HIV from concentrated populations to the general public through bridge populations such as sexual partners (UNAIDS 2002a).

The United Nations produced a consultative report on what UN agencies should do in response to the IDU-related epidemic of HIV/AIDS globally. The main findings of this report are:

- Needle and syringe programs are a component of a comprehensive package for HIV/AIDS prevention among injecting drug users.
- The response to HIV/AIDS should be strengthened within UNODC, and it has a responsibility to scale up activities on HIV/AIDS given its channels of communications to respective government entities and civil organizations. However, specific expertise on HIV/AIDS needs to be added to UNODC offices.
- WHO has little country capacity specific to HIV/AIDS among drug users, but has the most important role to play in prevention through training and capacity building.
- The country-level response is complex due to differences in the extent of the epidemic among IDUs; the characteristics of the drug users, national laws, legal provisions and policies towards IDUs; public opinion and stigmatization; the status of civil society organizations; and the technical capacities of UN offices in each country.

The report calls for development of country-specific strategies based on common country assessments. Two Central Asian countries (Kazakhstan and Uzbekistan) were included in the assessments made for this report (Kroll 2002).

The UN Interagency Group on Young People's Health Development and Protection seeks to establish a common agenda for programming on adolescent health and development (WHO, UNFPA, and UNICEF 1997). This is described as a rights-based approach involving agencies that concentrate on the health of young people. It focuses on advocacy for favorable policies; information, education, and communications strategies; providing adequate and confidential health, counseling, and other services for young people; research and analysis to evaluate program effects; capacity building and developing best practices; and ensuring the participation of young people in local strategy development. The core mechanisms for efforts in the region have involved joint work plans on peer education and life skills and Youth Friendly Services (UNAIDS 2002b). Examples of actions to date are:

- Peer education assessments, peer training workshops, and materials development
- Life skills education in several ECA countries, including Central Asia; analysis of out-of-school approaches to life skills training; and assessment of health promoting school programs, life skills, and peer education.
- Assessment and strategic planning on Youth Friendly Services.
- Social mobilization and advocacy training and strategy development.
- Rapid assessment and response (RAR) studies in several ECA countries in preparation for the development of grant applications to the Global Fund to Fight AIDS, TB, and Malaria.

In addition, UNICEF developed a Medium Term Strategic Plan (2002–2005) as an explicit priority for the agency. In conjunction with other core commitments (girls' education, integrated early childhood care and development, immunizations, health systems development, and child protection), four priority areas are identified for action:

- Prevention of HIV infection among young people (information, life skills, access to services, and safer behaviors);
- Prevention of Parent-to-Child transmission of HIV (PMTCT)
- Providing care for children and parents living with HIV;
- Ensuring protection, care and support for orphans and children in families vulnerable to HIV/AIDS.

In the context of both development and emergency responses, reforms are sought in terms of residential institutions, juvenile justice, community capacities to care for the most vulnerable young persons, and policy advocacy. UNICEF also supports the International Harm Reduction and Development Network (IHRD), which targets needle exchange, substitution therapy, and outreach to marginalized groups. UN involvement is in general weak in this field, but it has potential as emergency response, especially to very underserved minorities such as Roma. Directions for UNICEF include training on IDU programming, development of a common approach among agencies on advocacy, partnership development, focusing PMTCT targeted to IDUs or partners of IDUs through harm reduction networks, and funding pilot/model projects.

For infected young persons, strategies to meet their psychosocial needs as well as health, legal, and employment issues require a continuum of care approach; this should also include orphans of AIDS victims. As such projects are scaled up, it is recognized that greater government ownership is necessary. One particularly important emergency function supported by UNICEF was the Rapid Appraisal and Response research undertaken in several Central Asian countries. However, UNICEF policy is clear in that it will not take on the role of direct service provision. Rather, it could help to ensure supply and entry points to address young persons. It would not supply needles and syringes for exchange programs (UNICEF 2001 and 2002).

The 18 countries originally targeted for STI Task Force work in Eastern Europe in 1998 included the Central Asian countries of Kazakhstan, Kyrgyz Republic, Tajikistan, Turkmenistan, and Uzbekistan. The task force recognized the concurrent epidemics of STIs and unsafe sexual behavior as cofactors for HIV transmission, the issues of trafficking and increased use of intravenous drugs in the region, and the underlying adverse socio-economic factors leading to poverty, sex work, migration, human trafficking, and lack of social cohesion. Funding for the STI Task Force secretariat has been provided by DFID, OSI/Soros Foundation, USAID, WHO, and UNAIDS (WHO Europe 2002). The main recommendations of the STI Task Force involve:

- Increasing access and affordability of services for STIs;
- Humanizing existing STI services;
- Including STI programs in health reform processes, especially case management at the primary care level and strengthening STI services within reproductive health services;
- Reaching out to marginalized groups to insure access to STI/HIV prevention and care, with associated legal and environmental changes needed to implement this activity;
- Promoting knowledge and skills for safer sex, especially among youth.

USAID Regional Strategy.[37] USAID has been providing significant financial and technical support to control of communicable diseases, including HIV/AIDS, STIs, and TB, in Kazakhstan, Kyrgyz Republic, Tajikistan, and Uzbekistan. USAID recognizes the rapid rise in HIV incidence in Central Asia and the nature of the concentrated epidemic among highly vulnerable groups, especially IDUs, CSWs, migratory populations, and bridging populations. It has developed a strategic program designed to prevent drug use among vulnerable youth and to control HIV spread among high risk groups. Among other activities, USAID has been financing:

- Control of infectious diseases, including establishment of HIV/AIDS sentinel surveillance (but not STI surveillance), with assistance from CDC.
- The Drug Demand Reduction Program (DDRP) aims at changing attitudes and practices among vulnerable groups of population. The program is financed until

---

37. USAID (2002). *USAID's Strategy on HIV/AIDS Prevention in Central Asia 2002–2004.* Available at http://www.usaid.gov/our_work/global_health/aids/Countries/eande/caregion.html

the end of 2005, and is implemented by a consortium of five agencies led by the Soros Foundation Kazakhstan.

- The four partner organizations are Population Services International (PSI), AIDS Foundation East-West (AFEW), Internews and Akkord. DDRP includes five components: i) professional training; ii) youth; iii) prisoners and commercial sex workers iv) refugees, migrants, displaced persons, and v) activities aiming at policy development. While the project aims to cover all critical areas, limited funds do not allow reaching fully highly vulnerable and vulnerable groups. There is no harm reduction component to this project.
- Condom Social Marketing is implemented by PSI and aims at increasing demand and improve access to condoms at subsidized price.
- The CAPACITY project will focus on capacity building for implementation of grants from GFATM and other large grants. Activities will include training and developing institutions and networks in the CAR to provide technical backup for implementation of HIV/AIDS programs at the national and regional levels.

Certain aspects of harm reduction programs, such as HIV testing and counseling, treatment of tuberculosis and other opportunistic and concomitant infections, syndromic case management of sexually transmitted infections and other ancillary services are financed by USAID. However, the US Government funds are not used to purchase or distribute equipment used for injecting illegal drugs, nor is illicit drug use condoned. Community outreach about the risk of injecting drugs, sharing needles, and the need for HIV testing and counseling is supported. In addition, in conjunction with the US Centers for Disease Control and Prevention (CDC), substantial resources are devoted to HIV/AIDS surveillance system development, blood safety, infant mortality prevention, and epidemiological training.

CDC will implement second generation HIV surveillance in four of the Central Asian Republics, using WHO recommendations to improve collection, analysis, and use of data from highly vulnerable groups. This is what is known as sentinel surveillance, which focuses primarily on injecting drug users and their partners and overlapping risk groups such as CSWs. This depends on the availability of laboratory test kits, which now include oral testing technologies (OraSure; CDC 2003a). Laboratory development for confirmatory testing procedures as well as surveillance of drug resistance are also high priorities. These also address needs for assuring safe blood supplies in the target countries. In addition, behavioral surveillance for risk factor data will be supported, and policy changes based on these data can be recommended. CDC now recommends HIV testing to be incorporated into routine medical practice when dealing with high risk groups, and thus it is assumed that such recommendations will be incorporated into USAID program inputs.[38]

USAID also supports a regional research strategy to describe sexual and injection drug use networks in cities with highest HIV incidence (USAID 2003d). This helps to describe the extent of youth participation in the networks, the AIDS transmission routes and protective behaviors, and exposure by targeted groups to preventive measures.

---

38. USAID and Central Asia Republics (CAR) Centers for Disease Control and Prevention (CDC) (2003). Program for Infectious Disease Control.

DFID Project. DFID will provide about $12 million over a four-year period (2004–2008) to improve the response to HIV/AIDS in Central Asia. The regional DFID program will support an enhanced regional response and the national programs in four countries (Kazakhstan, Kyrgyz Republic, Tajikistan, Uzbekistan). The grant will: (i) provide flexible and responsive TA to support a harmonized approach in the region supporting the UN principles of one national body, one national program and one national monitoring system; (ii) directly support the implementation of national harm reduction programs building on the capacity of civil society and national systems; and (iii) effectively work with the World Bank on design and implementation of the proposed regional project ensuring alignment of efforts. The goal of the DFID funded intervention will be to contribute to the aversion of a generalized HIV epidemic in the Central Asia region. The purpose will be to ensure effective implementation of comprehensive, national HIV/AIDS programs.

The DFID regional HIV/AIDS intervention is fully consistent with DFID's regional strategy, where HIV/AIDS is identified as a priority area, and the overall DFID policy on HIV/AIDS, as encapsulated in the UK's "Call for Action" paper. The strategic approach emphasizes an appropriate balance between prevention, care and impact mitigation and the importance of a national response and political leadership. It recognizes the needs and rights of vulnerable groups and highlights the increasingly important role of treatment in national programs with a focus on increased access and equity of distribution.

The key pillars of the proposed DFID program will be:

- Assistance (TA) for effective coordination across the region in the development, implementation and monitoring of national HIV programs, including effective use of Global Funds;
- Direct support to implementation of national HIV programs through harm reduction in vulnerable groups (Kyrgyz Republic, Tajikistan, Uzbekistan); and
- Assistance (TA) to the proposed regional initiative to support priority civil society interventions (highly vulnerable groups, migration, drug and human trafficking).

The principles of implementation of the DFID grant will be:

- Harmonized approach under national leadership, working towards full alignment behind a single national program. The DFID project will not set up parallel systems.
- Supporting the UN 'Three Ones'
- Joint monitoring and evaluation missions supporting the national system
- Strengthening existing political commitment across the region
- Supporting the development of an effective civil society reflecting the needs of poor and vulnerable groups

DFID's grants at the country level will become available towards the end of 2004. Part of the DFID grant will co-finance with IDA the proposed Central Asia AIDS Project, which is expected to become effective in 2005.

Table 20. Regional Agreements in Central Asia

Regional Agreements	Objectives	Steering Committee	Management/ Implementation	Member countries/ Partner organizations
CIS AIDS Agreement Emergency action program among Commonwealth of Independent States (CIS) on counteracting the HIV/AIDS epidemic May 30, 2002.	Implementation of regional and national strategies for counteracting the epidemic and ensure their implementation with resources from national budgets and other sources, including international assistance.	Council of Heads of Government of CIS. Executive Committee of CIS for coordination of issues related to Program implementation. Yearly Program review by CIS Council on Cooperation in Public Health.	National focal points for implementation. Implementation of specific activities through ministries and agencies of CIS countries.	CIS states in CAR, except Turkmenistan (which has not endorsed the agreement).
Drug Control Agreement Memorandum of Understanding on drug control cooperation between the Governments of Central Asia countries and UNODC May 4, 1996.	Strengthening drug, crime and terrorism control measures through technical cooperation programs and projects.		Regional office based in Tashkent and country offices.	All countries in the region.
Central Asia AIDS Declaration Regional Conference on HIV/AIDS Almaty, May 16–18, 2001	Commitment to scale up national responses to HIV/AIDS.			Kazakhstan, Kyrgyz Republic, Tajikistan.Uzbekistan and Turkmenistan were not represented but pledged support.

Central Asian Interstate Commission on Sustainable Development (CA-ICSD) and Central Asia Regional Environmental Center (CAREC) Charter www.carec.kz	Preparation and implementation of an agenda and model to address priority environmental, social and economic problems by establishing partnerships between Governments and other sectors for development and implementation of the Central Asian Sustainable Development Strategy and Convention. Organization of training seminars to disseminate information through an expert network and establish an accessible database.	ICSD has a coordination and political role.	CAREC provides financial and technical support. CA Governments provide technical and institutional support. Private sector and international organizations will also participate in the project.	Kazakhstan, Kyrgyz Republic, Tajikistan, Turkmenistan and Uzbekistan. International organizations: ICSD, CAREC, UNECE, OSCE, UNCSD, UNDP, UNEP.
Central Asian Cooperation Organization(CACO) Regional Agreement February 2002.	Development of cooperation for exchange of information, economic co-operation, and long-term action to prepare join reports and broaden political, social and other ties	Elected chairman of the CACO. Council of Heads of State. Council of Prime Ministers. Council of Ministers of Foreign Affairs.	National coordinators for special tasks.	Signed by all CAR countries except Turkmenistan.
Central Asian Transboundary Biodiversity Project (GEF-funded).	Improvement and harmonization of national legal and regulatory frameworks and establishment of a trust fund that could finance long-term biodiversity conservation activities.	Regional Steering Committee includes members of National Steering Committees responsible for overall project and trans-national coordination National	Regional Project Implementation Unit in the Ministry of Environmental Protection of the Kyrgyz Republic Country PMUs in line ministries in each participating country.	Kazakhstan, Kyrgyz Republic, Uzbekistan.

(Continued)

Table 20. Regional Agreements in Central Asia (*Continued*)

Regional Agreements	Objectives	Steering Committee	Management/ Implementation	Member Countries/ Partner Organizations
	Improved regional coordination and support of a regional trans-national supervisory committee.	Steering Committee includes Ministry of Finance Sector Ministries State Environmental Agency Regional authorities scientific community NGOs		
Central Asian University				
1997: International Commission to plan the University		Single international institution, private and self-governing university	Board of Trustees also bears full responsibility for its overall direction and day-to-day management.	Kazakhstan, Kyrgyz Republic, and Tajikistan.
2000: International Treaty establishing the University signed by the Presidents of Kazakhstan, the Kyrgyz Republic and Tajikistan, and the Aga Khan, and ratified by the Parliaments of Kazakhstan, Kyrgyz Republic and Tajikistan		The Aga Khan is Chancellor of the University. Fully independent Board of Trustees governs the University and will have legal ownership of its physical plant and other assets. Board of Trustees comprises representatives of participating countries and from other countries.	Trustees name a Rector, who is responsible for recruiting Deans, faculty members, and staff, with all appointments to be confirmed by the Trustees acting as a group. The Rector is responsible to the Board of Trustees.	Other countries can join the treaty at any time. Funded by individual donors, private foundations, international corporations, international development agencies and national Governments in the developed world, with University's endowment of $15 million sponsored by the Aga Khan.
Several Water-related Treaties Syr Darya River Basin 1990s.		Interstate Water Coordination Commission	All treaties failed because of short-term unilateral planning and weakness of enforcement mechanisms of agreements, which created a mentality of non-compliance.	Kyrgyz Republic, Uzbekistan and Kazakhstan.

Stakeholder Analysis and Institutional Assessment

Stakeholders and Institutions

The Central Asia HIV/AIDS and TB Country Profiles identified stakeholders affected by the disease or having some intervention in this area; and the lack of capacity of organizations working on HIV/AIDS to operate effectively (Godinho and others 2004). The Country Profiles (2003) identified variable participation and poor institutional capacity in some countries. Further assessments were undertaken to take a closer look at the stakeholders and institutions involved on this issue, and make recommendations for improvements on stakeholder participation and institutional capacity (River and others 2003). This section of the report draws on international experience in discussing the value of stakeholder participation and assessing organizational capacity, and identifies more closely the needs, gaps and opportunities for stakeholder involvement and organizational development.

Internationally, the institutional performance required to successfully address HIV/AIDS has been identified as including a strong national political commitment at the highest level, multi-sectoral and multi-level responses, effective monitoring of the epidemic and risk behaviors, programs to sustain awareness aimed at both the general population and high risk groups, and programs that integrate prevention and care (UNAIDS 2001 and 2002). In order to be effective, country action needs to be implemented on a large scale.

As indicated in the policy analysis in the previous section, all five countries in Central Asia have recognized the impending danger of an HIV epidemic, and have recently approved national strategies and/or programs on HIV/AIDS. Governments have taken positive steps to modify legislation to include HIV/AIDS detection and introduce confidentiality provisions. The regional declaration signed by Central Asian Governments in 2001 is a major breakthrough in recognizing the problem.

Implementation of the approved HIV/AIDS strategies in Central Asia raises the following questions:

■ Is the infrastructure in place to act on these strategies?

■ Are all the necessary stakeholders involved?

■ Are the resources available or dedicated to fulfill the strategic priorities?

■ Are the organizations that will contribute to reducing the incidence or impact of HIV/AIDS at the necessary stage of capability and capacity development?

■ Are the institutions responsible for service delivery to high-risk groups able to achieve the coverage needed for adequate control of the epidemic's growth?

This section addresses the questions included in the box above. The study does not attempt to quantify or evaluate the current level of performance of organizations against their programs. The report is not an audit of stakeholders and systems. Rather it identifies the strengths and weaknesses of the program delivery against the stated strategies of each country. Where possible, the study has identified whether organizational resources are allocated in a manner that is consistent with country strategic directions, gaps in capacity, engagement with primary stakeholders and interagency collaboration. Firsthand information from those affected by HIV/AIDS should emerge from the focus groups being undertaken. This will assist in determining future directions for organizations and their services

The stakeholder analysis and institutional assessments were carried out on the basis of reviews of existing data and reports on HIV/AIDS in Central Asia, including country applications to the GFATM; and visits to Kazakhstan, Kyrgyz Republic, Tajikistan, and Uzbekistan, including meetings with government departments, local and international NGOs, and donors. In addition, the following studies have being carried out that add relevant information in this area:

■ Focus groups to obtain first-hand information from those with HIV/AIDS, and from those providing services have being carried out in Kazakhstan, and will be replicated in other Central Asian countries (Cercone and others, Forthcoming); and

■ Public opinion research in the Kyrgyz Republic to gain an insight into decision- and opinion-makers levels of awareness, knowledge, attitudes and practice (Felzer 2004).

The Need for Stakeholder Participation to control HIV/AIDS

HIV/AIDS is no respecter of the divisions between personal and public health for individuals, families, or communities. Nor does it respect the social and economic lines drawn between individual suffering, family and community impact, the impact on whole sectors of the population, and the social fabric and economy of a country. The government agencies established to deal with health, education, youth and social welfare, or economic planning and financial management often operate as separate "silos" with separate strategies, budgets, and lines of accountability. This doesn't work when dealing with HIV/AIDS. HIV/AIDS calls for coordination between agencies within government, and between the government, NGO and the private sectors. It also calls for collaboration between those affected by the disease and those with technical expertise about the disease. Involving stakeholders directly, whether people living with HIV, at risk groups or medical groups, and others involved in service delivery, leads to the development of better policies and programs. Ways in which this involvement can be achieved are described below. International experience has identified the combined importance of the following characteristics for HIV/AIDS programs to be effective (UNAIDS 2001 and 2002):

- Strong political commitment at the highest level (this ensures policies and funding to address the problem);
- Multi-sectoral approaches to prevention and care;
- Multi-level responses (at national, provincial, district and community levels);
- A combination of efforts aimed at the general population and focused on groups at high risk at the same time;
- Effective monitoring of the epidemic and risk behaviors, and dissemination of the findings both to improve policies and programs and to sustain awareness;
- Implementation on a large scale; and
- Integrated care and prevention.

The first four points indicate the need for multi-stakeholder and multi-sector involvement, and collaborative and coordinated approaches. This means in practice:

- Multi-sectoral approaches that work through horizontal integration/interconnections (for example, between government agencies, NGOs and donors) and vertical interconnections (for example, from the Prime Minister through to small community organizations who support those with HIV/AIDS or patients who can in turn support others).
- Involving those who are affected by HIV/AIDS to help design solutions, to help educate others, and to reduce stigmatization (UNAIDS 2001; Peddro 2001).
- Involving the variety of actors who know most about the disease, or are likely to be impacted by the disease. This is important for effectiveness in finding appropriate, relevant responses to either prevent or treat HIV/AIDS. It is also important for promoting allocative efficiency through appropriate targeting and better allocation of scarce resources while ensuring equity of access to services.[39]

---

39. Joshua L (2003). Social Insurance Technical Assistance Project [SITAP] Pensions workshop. Banja Luka, 7–8 July. World Bank Loan-funded project: Report No: 25672: Allocative efficiency means that the economy is doing the best job possible of satisfying unlimited wants and needs with limited resources — that is, of addressing the problem of scarcity. Efficiency in allocation is one dimension of efficiency. The term efficiency also has strong conceptual links with equity in that while efficiency focuses on financial and human inputs to support policy, equity can be delineated into equity in access, equity in capabilities and equity in outcomes. It is not always possible to achieve both efficiency and equity in equal measure, and therefore trade-offs are required between different types of efficiency and different types of equity. Institutional competencies and organizational arrangements are critical factors for ensuring that appropriate trade-offs between the different dimensions of efficiency and equity are made at appropriate junctures of policy formulation and policy implementation.

Participatory Decisionmaking

All of these factors reinforce an international trend away from directive, top-down decisionmaking systems to more participatory and democratic structures involving active relationships between stakeholders. These are based on developing trust relationships, sharing information and respecting the range of roles and skills needed to address HIV/AIDS. The pattern of the spread of the disease requires an open, engaging set of responses. This can be difficult, however, at the very time when cultural constraints and views about particular population groups support excluding, fear-based and punitive responses—often supported by lack of knowledge about the disease and how it spreads.

There is now constant international policy dialogue about the value and effectiveness of stakeholder involvement and participatory approaches. Approaches to participation that:

- foster genuine engagement between those who control resources and make decisions and those who are personally affected by HIV/AIDS;
- operate on a partnership basis;
- have advisory bodies;
- engage in high quality consultation where those consulted are listened to, and their views and experience taken on board and incorporated into policy, resource and service decisions;
- delegate control to those most appropriate to deliver services or information; and
- develop respectful and responsive care systems.[40]

These elements emerge as key to effectiveness in the design and delivery of HIV/AIDS programs. This is particularly important given the disease's lack of respect for social, economic and spatial boundaries, and cultural beliefs, and the personal and private nature of its transmission. Increasingly there is international experience of the lack of progress in dealing with HIV/AIDS if the non-participation route is taken (Burns and Morgan 2001).

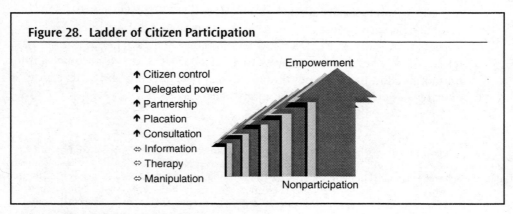

Figure 28. Ladder of Citizen Participation

↑ Citizen control
↑ Delegated power
↑ Partnership
↑ Placation
↑ Consultation
⇔ Information
⇔ Therapy
⇔ Manipulation

Empowerment

Nonparticipation

Source: Based on Arnstein (1969).

40. Based on literature addressing participatory approaches, including Arnstein (1969) and Nazurov, Rose, and Shelley (2000).

Stakeholders

This report refers to two main types of stakeholders: those most directly affected by HIV/AIDS, and those with a responsibility to respond to the HIV/AIDS epidemic through social, policy or service functions.

Primary stakeholders, are those most affected by HIV/AIDS. Given the characteristics of HIV/AIDS in Central Asia, they are: intravenous drug users (IDUs), commercial sex workers (CSWs), men having sex with men (MSM), those in prisons, young people, and migrants and refugees who, for poverty reasons often engage in risky activity such as commercial sex. For this first group and PLWHA, important issues are:

- how included or excluded they are from society,
- their levels of knowledge, awareness and practice (for prevention and treatment),
- opportunities to be listened to and understood,
- opportunities to participate in epidemic control and to contribute to service delivery planning, and
- safe and easy access to quality diagnosis and treatment.

Secondary stakeholders, include the organizations that represent national and international collective priorities for economic and social development, and voluntary commitment to addressing concerns. These stakeholders include government ministries, donors, international and national NGOs, and local communities.

The two sets of stakeholders are strongly inter-connected. The way in which they work together is fundamentally important, especially in a world that is increasingly moving away from autocratic, command and control styles of decisionmaking to greater participation and democracy. Because stakeholder participation involves organizations as well as individual citizens, the capacity of those organizations to operate effectively is of paramount importance. There is no single, patented way to ensure organizational capacity.[41] Improving capacity is also an ongoing process, but for addressing HIV/AIDS there are some key factors to take into account:

- Is there a strategy in place?
- Do the strategies of individual stakeholder organizations contribute to the overall HIV/AIDS strategy?
- Are adequate resources dedicated to achieve the strategies?
- Do the organizations have the structure, systems and skills to implement the strategy?
- Given the interdependent nature of responses to preventing or addressing HIV/AIDS, do the agencies have a collaborative approach to decisionmaking?
- Do the agencies have effective ways of engaging with those who are most affected by HIV/AIDS?

Because HIV/AIDS does not respect boundaries, effective multi-sectoral responses require the agencies involved to collaborate—and move beyond protecting the boundaries

---

41. There is a useful discussion around capacity building issues in CDRA, *Capacity Building: Myth or Reality,* 1994/1995, Annual Report at: www.cdra.org.za.

of their own organization. Although multi-sectoral collaboration to fight HIV/AIDS has emerged in the region lately, with assistance from UNAIDS and donors, it is at an initial stage and much needs to be done to improve such collaboration. Key elements of effective collaborative decisionmaking include: (i) that the joint activity between two or more agencies increases public value through working together in a strategic and results-focused manner; and (ii) that the processes stake out common ground, identify where territorial protection between agencies acts as a barrier to achieving the common good or public value, and often help correct misperceptions about the size and scope of conflicts.

Collaborative, interagency decisionmaking incorporates objective and subjective components. Objective components include: formal agreements at the executive level; personnel; budget allocations and resources assigned to collaborative tasks. Subjective components include: relevant individuals' expectations of others and competency at performing collaborative tasks. As a result it is important to have processes in place for ongoing collaboration (Bardach 1998).

Current Situation for Stakeholders and Organizations

Primary Stakeholder Population Groups. Tables 6 and 7 in the first section of this report show the main stakeholders for the four overlapping epidemics in Central Asia. While the relative sizes and dynamics of the different groups most at risk from HIV/AIDS vary between countries, they share many characteristics:[42]

- Intravenous drug use is widespread and increasing rapidly. Because the countries are on the drug route from Afghanistan, drugs are readily available.[43]
- Increasing numbers of women, girls and men are engaged in commercial sex work.
- Poverty and unemployment feeds the increase in drug use and prostitution.
- Many sex workers are engaged in the activity for relatively short periods, many returning to rural areas. This turnover makes safe-sex education, HIV/AIDS education and health monitoring difficult, and increases opportunities for disease to be spread into regions that lack the medical facilities of the cities.
- Everywhere among at risk groups the knowledge of measures to prevent the spread of HIV/AIDS is dangerously poor, and the use of condoms is correspondingly low.
- The low use of condoms, even by CSWs, and the use of dirty injecting equipment, reflects both a lack of awareness of the risks and also the costs. Injecting drugs is more often a social activity that involves sharing the drug and the equipment, adding to the risks of transmission.
- Prisons that are overcrowded are notoriously fertile ground for spreading HIV infection, and TB, as TB is widespread in the penitentiary system. The attention paid to this is relatively low in Central Asian countries, with most knowing little about the incidence of infected prisoners.

---

42. There is less information about primary stakeholders in Uzbekistan than other countries.

43. In Turkmenistan, local researchers found that the habit of smoking drugs instead of injecting protects drug users from HIV infection.

> *"The President will not speak openly about rates of AIDS in the country. But he will openly propose to fight drug use in the country".*
> **One of the Respondents in Uzbekistan**
>
> *"Kyrgyz Republic, a country which until recently few people even knew existed, is likely to become the first of the Former Soviet countries to scale up a variety of harm reductions services, including methadone maintenance treatment".*

The concerns that people have about being forcibly detained, discriminated against or ostracized can deter them from possessing condoms, using needle exchanges, or from seeking HIV testing or treatment for symptoms if there is an atmosphere of fear and punishment, rather than support for victims of the disease.

Despite a growing emphasis on coordinated regional responses, it is important that any HIV/AIDS initiative in Central Asia must continue to accommodate a cultural reluctance to confront HIV/AIDS. This shows itself most clearly in the fear-based or punitive approach to drug users. Historically, National HIV/AIDS centers in the former Soviet Union focused on mandatory mass screening, based on traditional "identify and control the carrier" approaches. In addition, human rights are neglected. Those living with HIV/AIDS were afraid to seek treatment, fearing government retribution. Similar concerns exist today and were quite openly acknowledged by respondents in their comments about constraints associated with confronting HIV/AIDS. Typical comments from Uzbekistan were:

> "Our police officers are telling everyone that I am HIV positive. After this I started having problems with my neighbors and friends"
>
> "I have a friend who is working in the local municipality. She told me that they are given lists of HIV-infected people who live in the district."
>
> "We do not know where to turn and who to talk to concerning this disease … not everyone should know but it is not easy; when you call an ambulance or go to the clinic you have to explain … people step aside, loudly express their opinions, including that all AIDS patients should be eliminated. It is frightening to hear… A support group should be established at the AIDS center and a hot line service…"

Combined with questions about the coverage of official statistics, these i support the view that the incidence of HIV/AIDS in these countries is under-r understated. While there have been some individual studies identifying t attitudes and practices of primary stakeholders, this has not been assessed. This is understandable given the relatively recent multi-stake HIV/AIDS. It also reflects the lack of accurate data on the actual num by HIV/AIDS. The work being undertaken by USAID, and CDC i help pinpoint more accurately where those living with HIV/A most helpful.

Country Commitment within the Region

Government responses to HIV/AIDS in the countries of Central Asia vary in their levels of commitment. For example in Kazakhstan the budget allocations do not appear to yet be following the strategic directions for HIV/AIDS. For the Kyrgyz Republic there are gaps in financial resource allocation. The concern with Tajikistan is that the country's financial situation is so dire that the HIV/AIDS strategy will remain a paper exercise. The assessments showed that interagency cooperation is improving. In some countries, the level of collaboration is more advanced, (for example, in Kazakhstan), then in others. However, current levels of collaboration are still inadequate to offer an effective response for epidemic control. Thus, processes that further interagency, inter-sectoral and regional collaboration become extremely important. Each country is assisted by significant donor input that is, to a certain extent, regionally coordinated. Tables 8 and 9 in the first section of this report, give some indication of the overall approaches being taken in terms of strategies/programs, coordination and donor input. Table 10 provides some indicative information about financial resources for HIV/AIDS.

Kazakhstan. In Kazakhstan there is recognition of the HIV/AIDS problem and the importance of a preventive approach. There is high level leadership in Kazakhstan, with buy-in from the Presidential Administration and Government. Changes to legislation for consistency will be important. Access to counseling for vulnerable groups is limited. There would be value in reinforcing and strengthening advocacy and education work to promote more understanding attitudes towards PLWHA in prisons, and among the Police towards IDUs and PLWHA. While "Trust Points" have been established, there appear to be significant issues with their location (and lack of sense of being a safe place to go to), and over the quality of their services. The Republican AIDS Center is understaffed and has insufficient funding to provide support, networking and assessment of quality standards. While there are a number of NGOs, locally based NGOs are often very slimly resourced, and quite fragile in their structure and operation. Many have not been operating for long and would have difficulty scaling up in their current state. They warrant continued and focused assistance and support.

Kyrgyz Republic. For the Kyrgyz Republic, a considerable achievement is the recognition of the importance of HIV/AIDS. There is high level leadership and buy-in from the [...] Administration and Government. The Kyrgyz Republic's willingness to [...] HIV epidemic when the first cases were identified can be considered [...] practice. However, the absence of a really coordinated state policy and [...] and programs for vulnerable people is a problem. The national [...] has been established but is still fragile in its operation. [...] of key government and NGO players have been well [...] easing expertise. Financial resources and technical [...] GO sector is relatively developed (20 in 2004) [...] ssociation of AIDS-service NGOs has been [...] DP, some NGOs appear to be quasi-NGO [...] ublic servants. There is concern about them [...] is also concern about areas of congestion by

Country Commitment within the Region

Government responses to HIV/AIDS in the countries of Central Asia vary in their levels of commitment. For example in Kazakhstan the budget allocations do not appear to yet be following the strategic directions for HIV/AIDS. For the Kyrgyz Republic there are gaps in financial resource allocation. The concern with Tajikistan is that the country's financial situation is so dire that the HIV/AIDS strategy will remain a paper exercise. The assessments showed that interagency cooperation is improving. In some countries, the level of collaboration is more advanced, (for example, in Kazakhstan), then in others. However, current levels of collaboration are still inadequate to offer an effective response for epidemic control. Thus, processes that further interagency, inter-sectoral and regional collaboration become extremely important. Each country is assisted by significant donor input that is, to a certain extent, regionally coordinated. Tables 8 and 9 in the first section of this report, give some indication of the overall approaches being taken in terms of strategies/programs, coordination and donor input. Table 10 provides some indicative information about financial resources for HIV/AIDS.

Kazakhstan. In Kazakhstan there is recognition of the HIV/AIDS problem and the importance of a preventive approach. There is high level leadership in Kazakhstan, with buy-in from the Presidential Administration and Government. Changes to legislation for consistency will be important. Access to counseling for vulnerable groups is limited. There would be value in reinforcing and strengthening advocacy and education work to promote more understanding attitudes towards PLWHA in prisons, and among the Police towards IDUs and PLWHA. While "Trust Points" have been established, there appear to be significant issues with their location (and lack of sense of being a safe place to go to), and over the quality of their services. The Republican AIDS Center is understaffed and has insufficient funding to provide support, networking and assessment of quality standards. While there are a number of NGOs, locally based NGOs are often very slimly resourced, and quite fragile in their structure and operation. Many have not been operating for long and would have difficulty scaling up in their current state. They warrant continued and focused assistance and support.

Kyrgyz Republic. For the Kyrgyz Republic, a considerable achievement is the recognition of the importance of HIV/AIDS. There is high level leadership and buy-in from the Presidential Administration and Government. The Kyrgyz Republic's willingness to respond to a potential HIV epidemic when the first cases were identified can be considered international best practice. However, the absence of a really coordinated state policy towards prevention programs and programs for vulnerable people is a problem. The national level coordination mechanism has been established but is still fragile in its operation. An important step is that the roles of key government and NGO players have been well defined, and each is active and with increasing expertise. Financial resources and technical assistance are major gaps. Although the NGO sector is relatively developed (20 in 2004) and has the potential for scaling up, and an Association of AIDS-service NGOs has been established in 2002 with support from UNDP, some NGOs appear to be quasi-NGO service providers set up and run by senior public servants. There is concern about them having preferred access to resources. There is also concern about areas of congestion by

> *"The President will not speak openly about rates of AIDS in the country. But he will openly propose to fight drug use in the country".*
> **One of the Respondents in Uzbekistan**
>
> *"Kyrgyz Republic, a country which until recently few people even knew existed, is likely to become the first of the Former Soviet countries to scale up a variety of harm reductions services, including methadone maintenance treatment".*

The concerns that people have about being forcibly detained, discriminated against or ostracized can deter them from possessing condoms, using needle exchanges, or from seeking HIV testing or treatment for symptoms if there is an atmosphere of fear and punishment, rather than support for victims of the disease.

Despite a growing emphasis on coordinated regional responses, it is important that any HIV/AIDS initiative in Central Asia must continue to accommodate a cultural reluctance to confront HIV/AIDS. This shows itself most clearly in the fear-based or punitive approach to drug users. Historically, National HIV/AIDS centers in the former Soviet Union focused on mandatory mass screening, based on traditional "identify and control the carrier" approaches. In addition, human rights are neglected. Those living with HIV/AIDS were afraid to seek treatment, fearing government retribution. Similar concerns exist today and were quite openly acknowledged by respondents in their comments about constraints associated with confronting HIV/AIDS. Typical comments from Uzbekistan were:

"Our police officers are telling everyone that I am HIV positive. After this I started having problems with my neighbors and friends"

"I have a friend who is working in the local municipality. She told me that they are given lists of HIV-infected people who live in the district."

"We do not know where to turn and who to talk to concerning this disease ... not every-one should know but it is not easy; when you call an ambulance or go to the clinic you have to explain ... people step aside, loudly express their opinions, including that all AIDS patients should be eliminated. It is frightening to hear ... A support group should be established at the AIDS center and a hot line service..."

Combined with questions about the coverage of official statistics, these influences support the view that the incidence of HIV/AIDS in these countries is under-reported and understated. While there have been some individual studies identifying the knowledge, attitudes and practices of primary stakeholders, this has not been comprehensively assessed. This is understandable given the relatively recent multi-stakeholder attention to HIV/AIDS. It also reflects the lack of accurate data on the actual numbers of people affected by HIV/AIDS. The work being undertaken by USAID, and CDC in Kazakhstan, which will help pinpoint more accurately where those living with HIV/AIDS are located, should be most helpful.

NGOs, international and government agencies in some areas, and gaps in other areas at national and rayon levels.[44]

Tajikistan. In Tajikistan, a National Program on AIDS adopted in 1997 and a second National STI/AIDS Program adopted in 2000 support a prevention and control approach. Unfortunately, serious financial constraints faced by the Government raise concerns about the implementation of the Programs. The UN Theme group appears to be an active and relatively effective mechanism for ensuring a coordinated approach among the main donors. They have prepared an integrated work plan that identifies areas of collaboration and serves to reduce overlap. However, the concern is that the GATFM funding will reduce any chance for Government finance to be provided.

Turkmenistan. Although Turkmenistan is rich in oil and natural gas, and has great potential for economic and social development, the majority of the population lives in poverty. Physical infrastructure and social services are extremely underdeveloped, and the country suffers from water shortage. Information about the status of HIV in Turkmenistan is limited with, officially, only two registered HIV cases. The Turkmen State News Service reported in 2001 that "AIDS is not a problem in Turkmenistan due to the success of the governmental anti-AIDS measures." However, the number of drug users has increased 4 fold in the period 1995–1997, according to official statistics. Turkmenistan has about 6,000 registered drug users, but UN agencies estimate that the real number is over 50,000, of which 15 percent would be IDUs. About 50 percent of those in prisons would be drug users. STIs have been increasing recently (7 fold for syphilis in the period 1992–98), and therefore the number of HIV cases is also expected to raise. The MoH recognizes that only about 30 percent of cases of syphilis and gonorrhea are identified by public services.

Although an HIV/AIDS Strategy has not yet been approved, the President signed a Law on prevention of HIV/AIDS in 1991, which has now been revised and is under consideration by the Parliament. The Government has adopted a National Program for HIV/AIDS (1999–2003). The plan is implemented with active assistance from the UN-AIDS Theme Group, but no monitoring and evaluation data on program results is available. The Government has a database on drug trafficking and drug use, but is reluctant to share any available data. UNODC carried out an HIV/AIDS Rapid Situation Assessment, but as has happened in other cases, the Government has not released the results of this study.

The Ministry of Health carries out HIV/AIDS education activities, but these have not been evaluated. The National AIDS Program includes plans to develop sentinel surveillance. UNAIDS has been supporting the introduction of information technology through the AIDS centers networks, but few computers are available at the Velayat level, and these centers do not have access to internet. Therefore, there is a lack of baseline studies, sentinel surveillance and behavior studies. In addition to modernizing monitoring by establishing sentinel surveillance, partners consider that it would be beneficial to measure the impact of IEC materials distributed in Ministry of Health, hospitals, outpatient centers, and schools

---

44. For example, there are 9 agencies working on IEC issues with young people and no agencies working on harm reduction with young people, or training of professionals in working with prisoners. There appear to be no agencies working on de-stigmatization through professional education providers

regarding HIV/AIDS and reproductive health issues. The Ministry of Health is planning to adopt the syndromic approach for STIs, although it is considered very expensive.

Only two international NGOs are working in Turkmenistan: Counterpart Consortium (funded by USAID) and MSF.

Uzbekistan. In Uzbekistan there appears to be no clear vision or coordination about which donors target which population or geographical location. There is oversubscription for IEC but, apparently, no finance for de-stigmatization programs—a major issue in Uzbekistan. While there are some dedicated NGOs in Uzbekistan, they are quite fragile and dependent on a few dedicated individuals. They require significant assistance to build capacity. Like the Kyrgyz Republic, there appear to be "real" NGOs, with others that exist in name only being supported by the Government. There is a significant question mark over the capability of the heath sector to deliver the needed services. There is also a lack of counselors and social workers. Uzbekistan and Kazakhstan both have difficulty in supporting the syndromic approach to STI treatment.[45]

Major Donors and International and National NGOs

Over the past five years several organizations have been providing financial and/or technical assistance to research and interventions to control HIV/AIDS, STIs, and TB in the region: UN agencies, bilateral agencies (such as USAID, KfW, and DFID), and international NGOs (such as the Soros Foundation/OSI and PSI) are assisting Central Asian Governments and NGOs, and are co-operating with each other. UNAIDS has provided significant assistance in the development of strategies. UNAIDS, UNICEF, UNFPA, USAID, and the Soros Foundation have been providing significant funding for HIV/AIDS prevention. However, the level of funding does not allow for the required scaling up of activities.

Kazakhstan. In Kazakhstan, all UN agencies, bilateral agencies such as USAID, and international NGOs such as Soros/OSI have been assisting the Government of Kazakhstan technically and financially in implementing HIV/AIDS prevention activities.

- UNAIDS has been assisting the government on policy issues.
- UN agencies finance HIV/AIDS prevention and healthy lifestyle programs.
- PSI has recently launched a program, with USAID support, for preventive maintenance of HIV-infection and venereal diseases.
- OSI/Soros Foundation is operating harm reduction programs and supports 31 "Trust Points."
- USAID and Centers for Disease Control (CDC) are assisting the development of sentinel surveillance, including training to improve data quality.

---

45. Syndromic management of STI: Treating a patient for all likely causes of a symptom or sign of an STI, rather than on the basis of a specific diagnosis (etiological management). Community-based syndromic management of STIs in the Mwanza, Tanzania, trial led to a 42 percent reduction in new HIV cases (Grosskurth and others 1995).

The government is actively working on improving the status and participation of NGOs and broader civil society. There is a proposed legislative change for government agencies to be able to contract NGOs to undertake work with vulnerable and highly vulnerable groups. Some initial moves have been taken and the Ministry of Health has recently contracted two NGOs (East to West and Equal to Equal) to discuss co-operation between AIDS Centers and NGOs.

Kyrgyz Republic. There is a rich combination of services with multiple players—Government, international donors, local NGOs, and International NGOs—operating a range of programs. The Kyrgyz Republic is actively promoting needle exchange programs to reduce infection. Public services and NGOs work with the highly vulnerable stakeholder groups such as IDUs, CSWs, and MSM. UN agencies, bilateral agencies and foundations such as Soros/OSI provide assistance to national agencies. Several government agencies closely co-operate with numerous national NGOs that cover several areas of drug abuse and HIV/AIDS prevention. These programs include:

- Socium is an NGO that works with drug addicts and provides medical assistance for IDUs along with psychological and social support.
- The NGO Sanitas Charity Fund deals with drug addiction among teenagers and provides treatment.
- Tais Plus is supported by UNDP to work on HIV/AIDS prevention for CSWs. Tais also carries out an IEC campaign. Supported by WHO, Oasis is an NGO that works with MSM by providing information on the prevention of HI/AIDS and legal support for MSM.
- WHO, the Republican Center for Health promotion and the Ministry of Education work on health promotion in schools, starting with four pilot projects.
- The army works closely with the NGO Bely Zhurav on an IEC program for young soldiers on preventing HIV/AIDS.
- The Ministry of Justice plans to allow the establishment of a methadone program in prisons. This is consistent with high levels of involvement of UN agencies, bilateral agencies and the Soros Foundation in drug use and HIV/AIDS prevention.
- The Soros Foundation/OSI have been working since 1999 with UNDP on harm reduction programs. These are now partially funded by USAID.
- UNICEF chairs the UN Theme Group, and has been operating a four-year program that includes a KAP baseline study of 15–19 year olds in five oblasts.
- UNICEF also assists NGOs working with street children.
- UNFPA works with the National AIDS Center addressing heterosexual transmission, estimated to be responsible for more than 20 percent of HIV positive cases. UNFPA works closely with other donors such as DFID and the Government of Netherlands to provide condoms for highly vulnerable stakeholders.
- UNHCR focuses on reproductive health and HIV/AIDS among refugee youth and supports NGO awareness campaigns among refugee youth.
- DFID is involved in providing substantial support for harm reduction programs.
- The Swiss Cooperation Office is providing some financial support for an information program on drug use.

Tajikistan. UNDP, UNICEF, and Soros have provided most of the technical and financial assistance for work with highly vulnerable groups in Tajikistan. For example,

- OSI/Soros Foundation and the Government jointly pay for volunteer costs, syringes and other supplies for Trust Points.
- UNICEF has been implementing a four-year program (2000–2004) that includes HIV/AIDS prevention activities with youth.
- The UN Theme group is active and organized in Tajikistan.
- A pilot to improve prison understanding and handling of prisoners with HIV/AIDS is being carried out. The Government has arranged for a study tour to Karaganda prison in Kazakhstan.

Turkmenistan. In Turkmenistan, the National Program for HIV/AIDS (1999–2003) aims to prevent the spread of HIV/AIDS through blood and sex. Program coordination is the responsibility of an Inter-Ministerial Task Force led by the Ministry of Health, National AIDS Center and the STIs Dispensary. In addition to the line ministries, the committee includes representatives from the Democratic Party of Turkmenistan, Women's Union, Youth Union, National Centre of Trade Unions, and the National Society of Red Crescent. The Program has been assisted by several UN agencies and other NGOs:

- The UN-AIDS Theme Group has supported the implementation of the AIDS National Program, including training of government staff and NGOs and education of young people.
- UNICEF has carried out estimates of the incidence of STIs and other diseases.
- UNODC carried out an HIV/AIDS Rapid Situation Assessment on trafficking and drug use in 2001.
- UNAIDS has provided syringes and bleach, including for prisons, and has been supporting the introduction of information technology particularly to assist with sentinel surveillance.
- UNFPA distributed more than 1 million condoms per year, and is working with the Army on reproductive health, contraception, STIs and urological diseases.
- UNICEF addresses issues of lifestyle, risk behavior, STI, HIV/AIDS and substance abuse in schools and youth clubs, and is carrying out a baseline assessment among youth.
- The Asian Development Bank has been assisting the UN-Theme Group on IEC, and training family doctors and nurses on counseling regarding HIV/AIDS.

Uzbekistan. In Uzbekistan, the UN Theme group is chaired by the World Bank and has the full support of the government. UNAIDS has worked closely with the government in the development of HIV/AIDS strategy.

- The Ministry of Health works closely with a range of UN and other donor agencies on the implementation of HIV/AIDS activities.
- UN agencies and USAID/CAR have been running mass media training and raising public awareness on drug related issues.

- ▓ UNICEF has been conducting an IEC strategy to raise awareness regarding drug abuse and safe sexual behavior.
- ▓ UNODC and the Government of Switzerland have been assisting the establishment of narcological health facilities for drug use treatment.
- ▓ USAID has been providing technical and financial support to HIV/AIDS prevention including upgrading the surveillance and lab system.
- ▓ OSI/Soros Foundation has been supporting the establishment of Trust Points, and works with the Ministry of Internal Affairs on the implementation of HIV/AIDS activities in prisons.
- ▓ OSI/Soros Foundation and IHRD are supporting the adoption of a policy of establishment of replacement therapy.
- ▓ PSI, with funding from USAID, has been implementing a condom social marketing campaign.
- ▓ Numerous NGOs work on HIV/AIDS in Uzbekistan, mainly funded by bilateral and international agencies. Among them:
- ▓ Kamolot works with youth,
- ▓ Sabokh and Istiqboli Avlod work with CSWs,
- ▓ Anti-AIDS works with MSMs, and
- ▓ Makhalla works with IDUs.

Assessment of Strengths and Gaps

During the last three or four years considerable steps have been taken by the region as a whole and more strongly by some individual countries to address the emerging HIV/AIDS problem. It has been said that Kyrgyz's willingness to respond to a potential HIV epidemic when the first cases were identified can be considered international best practice (Godinho and others 2004). The regional declaration signed by Central Asian governments in 2001 was a major breakthrough in recognizing the problem.

In undertaking initiatives, the governments of Central Asian countries were assisted by several multilateral and bilateral agencies. UNAIDS in particular has assisted with the development of country strategies. Other UN agencies and bilateral donors have supported specific streams of work and programs. They have frequently undertaken these initiatives with international NGOs, and increasingly, national NGOs where they exist. The level of national NGO development varies throughout the region. They are stronger in the Kyrgyz Republic and Kazakhstan, and weaker in Uzbekistan and Tajikistan.

The following discussion on strengths and weaknesses is based on looking at the situation and involvement of primary stakeholders, and the capacity of organizations that are secondary stakeholders. The analysis looked at the current strengths of development for HIV/AIDS prevention and control in Central Asian countries, and at obstacles to be surmounted in addressing the potential epidemic.[46] These are presented in Tables 21 and 22.

---

46. The analysis for this section of the report draws on country reports for Kazakhstan, Kyrgyz Republic, Tajikistan, and Uzbekistan.

Strengths. Key strengths that have emerged include:

■ The very *existence of Country Strategies*, including their multi-sectoral approach.
■ The particular value of *partnerships* developing between: donors and government agencies; government agencies and NGOs; donors, international NGOs and local NGOs; and regional government and NGOs. These provide the opportunity for different stakeholders to play to their strengths, reinforcing each other's roles, and providing a milieu for active learning from experience. The multiplicity of interagency coordination provides an excellent example of the potential in multi-stakeholder approaches, although those mechanisms are still weak and require support. National NGOs are clearly the lynchpin organizations in terms of relationships with vulnerable people—CSWs, IDUs, the homosexual communities, migrants, and young people.
■ The value of *piloting approaches*—such as the scheme in Kazakhstan focused on prisoners with HIV/AIDS or the MRT program in the prisons of Kyrgyz Republic— as long as lessons are actively learned from the pilot, and the questions (and answers) of ongoing ownership and sustainable funding are identified.
■ *Initial funding available* from UN agencies, and bilateral agencies for 5 countries and GFATM for Kazakhstan, Kyrgyz Republic, Tajikistan, and Uzbekistan allows to implement epidemic control interventions in the immediate future. However, funding levels would not allow to achieve high coverage of target groups with necessary services.
■ The value of planned, medium to long term *involvement of international agencies and donors* to help provide continuity and plan for sustainability, particularly in skills and funding.
■ The value of *multiple donors in the field*. This is particularly useful when donors and international NGOs operate in several Central Asian countries, do not overlap their funding programs, and provide the opportunity for an interconnected approach, and active contribution to capacity building. The combined assistance that USAID-CDC have provided to the development of surveillance systems in the region is one example. The USAID-PSI, and national NGOs working on social marketing and peer education by young people is another example. The UNDP support of Tais, an NGO working with CSWs in the Kyrgyz Republic is yet another.
■ The importance of supporting the *development of fledgling national NGOs* because they are the key "bridging" agencies between vulnerable populations, more formal agencies and society in general.[47] For example, in Uzbekistan, Sabokh, and Tiklal work with CSWs, Anti-AIDS works with MSMs and Mahala work with IDUs. In the Kyrgyz Republic, Oasis works with MSMs, and Socium works with drug addicts providing medical services and social support. In Kazakhstan, the Ministry of Health has contracted Equal to Equal working with those affected by HIV/AIDS.
■ The *opportunity to identify good practice and the opportunity to learn from examples of good practice within the region*. One example of this is the Uzbek government study tour to Karaganda prison in Kazakhstan to learn from the prison program with HIV/AIDS and IDUs.

---

47. The longest standing national NGO in Central Asia seems to have started in 1998.

These positive attributes provide the framework and some examples of developing capability. As practitioners in each of the countries have identified, there is still some distance to travel within a possibly short timeframe. Some possibilities for development emerge from the following presentation of weaknesses and gaps.

Weaknesses. This report has drawn on existing information about primary stakeholders—those most affected by HIV/AIDS. The information has shown limitations in terms of information about the knowledge, attitudes and practice (KAP) of those most affected by HIV/AIDS and by young people. In terms of the ability of those most affected by HIV/AIDS—including those living with HIV/AIDS—to be heard, understood, feel safe and participate in decisionmaking and policy setting, there is considerable work to be done. Preliminary information has identified consistent discrimination from the police. The importance of NGOs as life-lines—places that can provide a safe environment and practical information—was highlighted. Combined with early initial indications about lack of access to services, the role of NGOs becomes even more important. But there is much yet to be done before there is a comprehensive and focused approach. Before effective, meaningful action can happen resources are needed to implement each country strategy.

Weaknesses and Gaps. The weaknesses of the response to HIV/AIDS across the region include:

- *National (or regional) budgets often do not automatically or systematically follow the strategic directions and priorities to control the HIV/AIDS epidemic.* This can include the lack of a mechanism for ensuring the flow of resources to relevant agencies, and can become a major obstacle to building organizational capacity, and deliver appropriate programs. As examples:
  - While Kazakhstan budgets a reasonable amount of money, it does not execute the budget so that AIDS services are forced to operate mostly on grants from donor agencies.
  - In Tajikistan the concern with funding is fundamental—the HIV/AIDS strategy there is at risk of becoming a paper exercise because the government is in such dire financial straits and without adequate donor assistance will not be able to solve the problem over the next several years.
  - In Kazakhstan and the Kyrgyz Republic several government agencies that are key for implementing the HIV/AIDS strategy are insufficiently funded to develop policy, provide services or hire and train staff.
  - The Kazak Republican AIDS Center cannot provide the services it is mandated for, and the Kazak Ministry of Health has only one staff member dedicated to policy development and policy coordination in the area of HIV/AIDS.
  - In the Kyrgyz Republic the Ministry of Justice (prisons) and the Center for Health Promotion are very slimly funded and the National Blood Center is under-resourced.
  - In Uzbekistan the Ministry of Health has the mandate for leadership on HIV/AIDS but not the resources.
  - The prison system needs are ignored in almost all countries and almost no assistance is rendered to prisoners, who belong to the highly vulnerable groups.

▓ *The relatively recent development of country strategies and multilateral approaches.*
It takes time to develop structures, systems and ways of operating collaboratively.
These difficulties become evident through territory protection between agencies, a
lack of clear roles in relation to the strategy and a lack of formal or informal ways
of collaborating. For example, in Kazakhstan, Kyrgyz Republic and Uzbekistan,
the Republican AIDS Center, STIs Dispensaries, Narcology Services and/or TB
institutes have weak and unconstructive linkages even after the establishment of
the CCM and receiving grants from the GFATM. In the Kyrgyz Republic, the
AIDS Centers have not been participating in the review of the country's Sanitary-
Epidemiological services despite the fact that restructuring may have a significant
impact on them.

▓ *A clash or lack of shared attitudes, beliefs and values.* Conflicting approaches by key
providers produce barriers to implementing the strategy. Region wide the punitive
approach taken by the police toward IDUs and CSWs is a major problem. Police
harassment of IDUs around Trust Points destroys the ability of these services to
provide effective services to high-risk groups and makes them unsafe places to go
near, removing the very trust they are expected to foster.

▓ *The early stages of donor coordination.* Donor coordination is notoriously difficult
to "get right." This is seen in patchy coverage by donors and overlaps and may be
the result of lack of clarity, or negotiation, of roles and lack of explicit, planned linking with the country strategy. For example, there appear to be multiple sources of
funding for Information, Education and Communication (IEC) programs in
Uzbekistan and the Kyrgyz Republic, but in this latter country there is no donor
financing for developing teaching, material on HIV/AIDS for young people. In
Tajikistan and Uzbekistan there is a lack of funding for de-stigmatization programs
or education.

▓ *Organizations not in place, or lack of readiness of agencies to scale up quickly.* There
are several examples of this, particularly AIDS Centers and Trust Points in several
countries. The Kyrgyz Republican Center for Public Health was established in 2002
and is so poorly funded it probably cannot contribute to HIV/AIDS work over the
next 5 years. The agency operates on grants rather than core government funding.
Tajikistan requires a major focus on all systems and structures.

▓ *Human resource development issues.* Across the region there is a shortage of counselors. Services requiring attention in terms of skills development include: the
police, prisons, TB and AIDS agencies and Trust Points. Tajikistan requires special
attention across the board.

▓ *Service availability and quality.* The focus here is on unreliable service quality and
gaps in service provision. Trust Points that were established in Kazakhstan, Kyrgyz
Republic, Tajikistan, and Uzbekistan emerge as being highly variable in their service
quality and coverage.[48] There are accessibility issues, personal safety issues and
issues of staff skills. In the Kyrgyz Republic the National Blood Transfusion Center
cannot provide a guarantee of a safe blood supply throughout the country. The
provision of a safe medical blood supply is an essential ingredient for reducing the

---

48. The results from focus groups being undertaken should provide useful information on these issues.

spread of HIV/AIDS. This is a question that is best addressed through a technical assessment of current capability, skill and equipment across the region.

- ▨ *The fragility of fledgling national NGOs.* National NGOs are the life-link for highly vulnerable groups, people with HIV/AIDS and for their families. Almost always those agencies find it difficult to gain resources for operating and to have the status in society to influence policy directions, perhaps because they work directly with clients who are shunned by society. The services can then become reliant on the commitment, skill and energy of key individuals who can "burn out" after a short time.

Organizational capacity building issues for national NGOs include the length of time it takes an organization to develop when they have difficulty in fundraising; are dealing with culturally sensitive issues; need to develop their skills; have difficulty influencing policy; and need to put resources into coordination with other NGOs and service providers.

For historical reasons the Central Asian region shows a strong dependency of national NGOs on international donors. There can be fierce competition among NGOs for financing. Currently there are few national or regional coordinating mechanisms and there is little legal capacity for national NGOs to operate as true partners, or to be contracted by government agencies. The legislative changes planned for Kazakhstan, and the high standing of the Association of NGOs in the Kyrgyz Republic, are very positive examples to build on.

- ▨ *Differences between countries' ability to fund AIDS programs in the region.* For example, Tajikistan has an economic crisis. The Kyrgyz Republic has implemented many steps for addressing HIV/AIDS effectively but has a slimmer national resource base than Kazakhstan.
- ▨ *The potential impact that an increased incidence of HIV/AIDS could have on the economies of the region have yet to be assessed.* Stakeholders identified that modeling to assess the economic impact of HIV/AIDS on the region's economies could serve to focus even greater attention on the importance of containing the epidemic.

Recommendations

In terms of stakeholder involvement and organizational strengthening, primary stakeholders should ideally be able to influence the policies and practices of those agencies delivering services. For this, their voices need to be heard and respected, their safety ensured, and their expertise incorporated through participating in service planning and decisionmaking; and influencing the refinement of policies emerging from the country HIV/AIDS strategies.

The organizations that form the secondary stakeholders are the actors that will bring alive the implementation of country strategies for HIV/AIDS. Their organizational strategies need to reinforce and be consistent with country HIV/AIDS strategies. They need, in turn, the resources to implement the country strategy, and the organizational structures and skills to deliver high quality services on the required scale. They also need the mandate to collaborate with, or form partnerships with each other. Healthy national NGOs are critically important for country strategies to be implemented effectively. They develop trust and credibility with those affected by HIV/AIDS. Actively developing high quality practice by learning from each other can be powerful in speeding up the capacity for organizations to scale up their activities.

■ *For Regional Coordination.* It would be highly desirable to have the resources for implementing country strategies allocated in a manner that builds interagency collaboration, and regional coordination and collaboration. Such regional coordination could focus on:

● Building partnerships between the governments and critical institutions across the countries of the region (for example, the Ministry of Health, AIDS Centers, Trust Points, NGOs, Prisons) that will allow for the open exchange of ideas, policies and best practices.

● Creating and developing regional capacity in:

—technical areas (such as HIV/AIDS surveillance, safe blood supply, drug trafficking control, prison systems improvement),

—critical human resource development for adequate HIV/AIDS service provision, such as counseling and social work,

—exchange of high quality practice and learning lessons from experience,

—NGO sector development and collaboration, and

—Building connections in handling the drug epidemic and in the integration of HIV/AIDS, TB and STIs.

● Using every step to build understanding, ownership, leadership and championship in dealing with HIV/AIDS.

■ *For Governments*

● Assessing and developing organizational skill and capability in areas which are currently weak such as: social work, counseling, the knowledge, attitudes and behavior (KAP) of the police towards CSWs and IDUs; education in schools and prison programs with IDU prisoners.

● Building stronger connections between priorities and funding flows—country budgets and donor budgets.

● Using the multi-sector roundtables in each country to:

—foster the removal of overlaps and the filling of gaps in funding and interventions,

—share information about lessons learned and high quality practice within countries.

● Developing quick turn-around monitoring and evaluation of policies, and programs—as well as starting the process of longer term evaluations.

● Focusing on assessing the current state of systems and institutions for, surveillance and service provision.

● With NGOs, developing effective approaches for incorporating the experiences of those groups most affected by HIV/AIDS into policy development, and program design and delivery.

■ *For the World Bank*

● Work with governments, and UNAIDS and donors to facilitate increased advocacy , multi-sectoral coordination, and the development of a regional partnership for early prevention and control of HIV/AIDS. Specifically the Bank could contribute to documenting success stories and developing mechanisms for adequate dissemination of best practices within the Central Asian Region and beyond. Success stories could be built around:

—policy development and implementation,

—service provision (modality, type of organization, form of delivery, quality of services),

—organizational development structures and systems, and

—human resources capability development.

● Work with governments on systems for ensuring that budget allocations to government departments and NGOs are consistent with the country HIV/AIDS strategies.

● Work with governments, other donors and NGOs to identify the most effective/efficient ways of delivering key services, for example investigating the effectiveness of Trust Points. It could be useful to select a few Trust Points that are fostering high quality practice to clients and to identify national NGOs undertaking a similar role, using them as examples to learn from. (It would be particularly relevant to involve Akims and other relevant primary health care services.)

● Work with governments, other donors and NGOs to define more specifically the service and resource allocation gaps and overlaps in relation to strategic priorities.

● Work with other donors, national governments and NGOs to develop effective, quick turnaround, monitoring and evaluation tools for assessing organizational improvement.

▩ *For International partners and NGOs.* National NGOs have emerged clearly as the agencies that are closest to the primary stakeholders most affected by HIV/AIDS. Effective NGOs develop trust with those affected by HIV/AIDS because they deliver relevant services, respect the confidentiality of clients and provide the support required by clients. They play a significant bridging role. International NGOs, in turn, provide the support to local NGOs in terms of training and resources, and act as a bridge between national NGOs, donors and government. These roles are well recognized and supported. They deserve greater and more focused support. It is recommended that UN agencies and international partners work with donors, governments and local NGOs on:

● Any further legislative changes to encourage and support NGO participation in effective service provision to high risk groups.

● The specific areas of assistance that NGOs require to ensure strong organizations, and effective, consistent and reliable high quality service delivery. Examples for organizational strengthening include: management and leadership skills, succession planning, and fundraising for continuity and security of service delivery. Examples for high quality service delivery include: specific skill requirements for counseling, advocacy, coordination and collaboration.

● Identifying funding streams within government and from donors to support the implementation of the plans developed for strengthening NGOs.

● Developing best practice models of the high quality and pioneering support work being undertaken by international NGOs and donors with national NGOs.

Table 21. Strengths On Which to Build for Addressing HIV/AIDS

Strengths	Country- or Region-specific Issues
▦ Country strategies based on a multi-sectoral approach	▦ Tajikistan the UN Theme group appears to be an active and relatively effective mechanism. Fledgling interagency coordination committee beginning to operate well.
▦ There is value where partnerships have developed and are developing between: donors and government agencies; government agencies and NGOs, donors, international NGOs and local NGOs; regional government and NGOs	▦ Kyrgyz Republic and Kazakhstan, high level ownership from deputy Prime Minister, but weak engagement of various sectors due to lack of resources.
▦ Useful to have piloted approaches	▦ Kyrgyz Republic's multi-party involvement is working well where a relationship of trust has developed between national NGOs, international NGOs and Government departments.
	▦ Prison pilot in Kazakhstan involving Soros and Ministry of Interior.
▦ There is value in the long term involvement of international agencies and donors	▦ The ability to transfer knowledge from one country experience to another and to foster learning between countries both within the region and outside the region.
▦ There is value when there are several donors in the field. There is particular value when donors and international NGOs operate in several CAR countries and provide the opportunity for an inter-connected approach, and active contribution to capacity building.	▦ Significant consistency when one can see UNAIDS, Soros/OSI, PSI, and others working together across the region, especially as they bring experience and expertise from their program involvement in other countries—either parts of eastern Europe (PSI turns to Russia as a bench mark) or in Africa.
▦ Fledgling development and involvement of NGOs	▦ Stronger capability of local NGOs in Kyrgyz Republic with several instances. Examples of highly constructive NGOs in Uzbekistan.
▦ The value of those NGOs who work closely with affected populations—CSWs, IDUs, prison staff particularly in terms of trust relationships developing and the NGOs ability to identify needs and deliver services and support that is culturally relevant, and effective.	▦ Uzbekistan and Kyrgyz Republic have several local NGOs working on HIV/AIDS. For example in Uzbekistan Kamalot work with youth; Sabokh and Tiklal Avlot work with CSWs; Anti-AIDS work with MSMs; and Mahal work with IDUs. Using one national NGO that works with MSM as an example, they have developed a large pool of volunteer MSMs that help to disseminate the information as well as outreach to new MSMs. They have developed significant trust among MSMs and could reach new groups and expand coverage.
▦ The opportunity to identify good practice.	▦ Kyrgyz Republic in terms of leadership and multi-sectoral team.
▦ The opportunity to learn from examples of good practice within the region.	▦ Uzbekistan—prisons and medical staff very interested in changing the rules and attitudes and providing better.
▦ Ownership taken by some government agencies.	▦ Tajikistan—a prison pilot on HIV/AIDS prevention and services where the government has arranged for staff to visit the Karaganda prison operation in Kazakhstan.
	▦ Kazakhstan Republican AIDS Center labs, and lab technical skills used by region.

Table 22. Obstacles to Organizational Development in Addressing HIV/AIDS

Weaknesses and Gaps	Country- or Region-specific
▪ Budget does not follow strategy	▪ Tajikistan—plans remain mainly paper exercises because the national budget is so constrained.
▪ Government strategic commitments not fulfilled by budgetary allocations	▪ Kazakhstan—Republican AIDS Center has insufficient funding for operations eg travel, networking, providing support, ability to assess standards, Center cannot employ PR/communications, psychologist or sociologist staff because of salary levels; Ministry of Health has only 1 staff member/position dedicated to strategy and policy development. Uzbekistan—Ministry of Health has mandate but no other strengths or resources in relation to HIV/AIDS; Ministry of Higher Education and teacher training organizations lack resources. significant variation in regional allocation of funds; essentially dependent on leadership of regional Akim rather than strategy and its implementation being structured with funding as part of the system.
▪ Resources not following either strategic priorities or mandates and the consequent difficulties in developing institutional capability and capacity.	
▪ No clear mechanisms for ensuring the flow of resources to relevant agencies to adequately implement strategies, for example resources availability in regions or oblasts	
▪ Newness of strategies and multi-sectoral approach	▪ Kyrgyz Republic—lack of budget resources; National Blood Transfusion Center probably under-funded; no teaching material for reducing youth vulnerability—overlooked in donor financing; AIDS center funding low. The Ministry of Justice for prison work and the Center for Health Promotion have a very low funding base.
▪ The relative newness of country strategies and a multi-sectoral approach to planning and decision-making. Becomes evident through:	▪ Kazakhstan—TB Center and AIDS Republican Center weak linkages when strong linkages important; narcology centers role and function not clear in national strategy of GATFM application. There is a network of narcology centers that could offer services to IDUs.
● 'territory' protection, and operating in 'silos',	▪ Uzbekistan—congestion of donor funding around IEC, gaps in funding support for de-stigmatisation programs.
● lack of shared resources,	
● lack of clear roles in strategies or GATFM proposals, and	
▪ lack of formal or informal approaches to collaborative decisionmaking	▪ Kyrgyz Republic—low political leadership in Ministry of Health for inter-sectoral coordination; uncertainty re involvement of Ministry of Justice in GATFM; restructuring of Sanitary-Epidemiological services brings uncertainty re AIDS centers—no communication over this; Republican Center for Health Promotion has not contributed to HIV/AIDS strategy and probably under-resourced to play significant role—no outreach to villages.
▪ Mixed messages or lack of shared values Conflicting approaches by key providers provides a major barrier to implementation of strategy through service provisions	▪ Uzbekistan—punitive approach by police to IDUs and CSWs potentially cancelling out, or creating obstacles, for the supportive work being undertaken by NGOs, some Trust Points and the donor community.

Table 22.   Obstacles to Organizational Development in Addressing HIV/AIDS (*Continued*)

Weaknesses and Gaps	Country- or Region-specific
■ Donor coordination just beginning—requires reinforcement and collaborative approaches for alignment with country strategies. This is seen in: ◆ Patchy donor financing; ◆ Uncertainty regarding roles, ◆ Uncertainty regarding common goals and how to achieve common goals together ◆ **Organizational Structures** ◆ Structures not in place, and the relatively recent establishment of some state agencies ◆ Lack of readiness of Trust Points (TPs) ◆ Lack of readiness of agencies to scale up quickly	■ Kazakhstan—police around Trust Points harassing and arresting. This point was raised consistently by national NGOs and international NGOs. It was also raised by government personnel and staff of Trust Points who are frustrated in not being able to do their work. ■ Tajikistan—Police do not understand harm reduction; harassment of IDUs and CSWs; lack of support for syndromic approach. ■ Kyrgyz Republic—teaching material for reducing youth vulnerability—overlooked in donor financing. ■ Multiple funding for IEC in Uzbekistan and Kyrgyz Republic. ■ Tajikistan and Uzbekistan—lack of funding for de-stigmatisation. ■ Throughout the regions TPs are not adequately developed and lack the resources and mix of staff skills to deliver adequate services. ■ In all countries, with the exception of Kyrgyz Republic, STI services are provided in an out-model fashion and are unable to respond to new demands. ■ Throughout the region the NGO capacity is weak. Although they are more developed in some countries, they are not in a position to be scaled-up and provide adequate coverage of services for high risk groups. ■ Kazakhstan—Republican AIDS Center insufficient resources. ■ Uzbekistan Institute of Health—good infrastructure but insufficient operational budget and staff with limited training. ■ Uzbekistan—Trust Points (TPs) established in 2000. ■ Kyrgyz Republic—Republican Center for Public Health established in 2002.

■ **Human resources development**

■ Skill shortages

■ Salary levels

- ▨ Kazakhstan—TPs not ready to scale up across the country—may be poorly located, poorly resourced from regional budgets.
- ▨ Tajikistan—significant, large-scale capacity building (structures, systems, skills development) required for majority of government agencies dealing with HIV/AIDS.
- ▨ Kazakhstan—lack of counsellors; and clinical and inter-personal skills of staff; lack of skilled teachers for HIV/AIDS education in schools; low salary levels making it difficult for Republican AIDS Center to recruit PR staff, sociologists and counsellors.
- ▨ Across region—lack of counsellors and staff who can provide social support.
- ▨ Across region—peer education. International NGOs noted that peer education is time-consuming to develop and implement.
- ▨ Lack of skilled staff across region in police and prison service with the skill and understanding of HIV/AIDS prevention and treatment to deal effectively with vulnerable groups and operate in a manner that is consistent with the country's HIV/AIDS strategy.
- ▨ Skills needed to develop common strategies between those agencies such as TB and AIDS agencies that are not co-operating with each other for the benefit of vulnerable groups and the population at large.
- ▨ Skills in educators/teachers on HIV/AIDS prevention, treatment.
- ▨ Tajikistan—skill development required in blood safety and surveillance, monitoring and evaluation skills for surveillance network, skills in HIV/AIDS prevention and treatment for government staff especially HIV focal points.

■ **Service availability and quality**

■ Unreliable service quality

■ Gaps in services

- ▨ Kazakhstan—variability of Trust Points around the country, quality issues around those that are operating (for example, service quality, location, safety).
- ▨ Kyrgyz Republic—lack of budget resources; National Blood Transfusion Center can't provide coverage of safe blood supply; lack of labs in prisons and unwillingness to use public labs.
- ▨ Tajikistan—see organizational structures above.

■ **Fragility of Local NGO Development**

■ Length of time it takes for NGOs to develop, especially when dealing with culturally sensitive issues

■ Many local NGOs focusing on HIV/AIDS have been operating for a short time

- ▨ Kazakhstan—interesting feedback from UNFPA on taking 4–6 years to develop rurally-based, local NGOs to deal with reproductive health issues effectively; PSI made similar comments on the time it takes to support/foster local community based organizations (CBOs) and NGOs—identifies the importance of building and supporting existing national NGOs.

(Continued)

Table 22. Obstacles to Organizational Development in Addressing HIV/AIDS (*Continued*)

Weaknesses and Gaps	Country- or Region-specific
▪ Relatively few national NGOs or community-based organizations (CBOs) ▪ Difficulty in raising funding ▪ Given the scale of the problem, few CBOs or local NGOs working with those affected by HIV/AIDS	▪ Kazakhstan—reliance on international donor input referred to in a recent study of NGOs in Kazakhstan (UNDP 2002). ▪ Tajikistan—while there are 1200 NGOs registered, in the country true capacity in the NGO sector is very limited—fierce competition for international donor funding because of lack of local funding sources. ▪ Not certain about the true status of some NGOs in Kyrgyz Republic and Uzbekistan—some have been established by government servants working in the HIV/AIDS arena as the funding has become available. ▪ The fundraising capacity of many national NGOs is very weak—noticeable in all CAR countries. ▪ There is often heavy reliance on international donors for funding. ▪ Little legal capacity for governments in CAR to contract with NGOs—although this is changing in Kazakhstan. ▪ The difficulties in assessing the numbers of "at risk" populations and the difficulties in providing services given the transient nature of street children, internal migrants (rural to urban and back again), refugees from other countries, and of CSWs—although work is being undertaken by USAID and CDC to identify the best ways of identifying at risk groups. The transience makes it difficult for NGOs to focus their work. It emphasises the importance of the trust relationships that can exist between NGOs and affected populations when there are effective operations.
▪ Few national or regional NGO coordinating mechanisms	▪ Useful to build on the initiatives in Kazakhstan to alter legislation for government contracting with NGOs, to support the fledgling approach to national-level NGO coordination, and to build on the NGO Association in Kyrgyz Republic which appears to play an effective advocacy role re HIV/AIDS.
▪ Unclear role of private sector ▪ Apparent invisibility of the private sector.	▪ NGO networks are at different stages of development in CAR countries. Generally, in all republics NGOs have failed to develop strong networks or a common platform for advocating to government, donors and international NGOs. ▪ In most countries visited there was no evidence provided of private sector involvement in HIV/AIDS issues. National strategies largely failed to address their possible role and try to involve the private sector in coordinated efforts to fight the HIV/AIDS epidemic.

Central Asia HIV/AIDS Communication and Participation Plan

Opportunities

▓ A "manageable" problem if dealt with in a rapid, open and efficient manner, as HIV is currently concentrated in clearly identified and clustered populations.

▓ Low prevalence rates across the region, although underreporting is rampant.

▓ Public services that could respond swiftly to a multi-sectoral approach, if a political mandate is obtained.

▓ A reasonably educated youth that may benefit from relevant preventive information.

▓ Entrepreneurial energy and high volunteerism, important for promoting counseling, social marketing, peer education activities, etc.

▓ Region culturally open to early action on drug control and prevention of HIV/AIDS.

▓ Engagement of international donors, multilateral and bilateral organizations, currently implementing targeted interventions with high-risk groups.

Obstacles

▓ Lack of public understanding of the social and financial costs resulting from the combination of increased drug consumption and the presence of HIV in the region, particularly among the young and/or economically-productive populations.

▓ Absence of political will, translated into negligible public funds for prevention, diagnosis, counseling and treatment of HIV/AIDS.

▓ Stigma and a legislation that criminalizes high-risk behaviors (sex-workers, IV drug-users, homosexuals, and so forth).

▓ Lack of information, particularly among vulnerable youth, about self-risk assessment, resulting in social denial of who is at risk.

▓ Erosion of social incentives and individual expectations among the vulnerable youth, which increases high-risk behaviors.

▓ Medical groups who will see their influence, resources and power diminished, as their mandate to deal with HIV/AIDS will be shared with others.

▓ Nascent civil society with incipient demand-creation mechanisms.

▓ Insufficient social pressure for accessible quality public health services.

While contextual barriers and opportunities will determine the scope and reach of national programs in the region, the urgency to increase public awareness cannot be over-stated. As the epidemic is still largely contained within clearly identified groups, this is the time to educate and inform about preventive behaviors, reduce vulnerability by introducing self-risk assessment mechanisms, and develop community responses to discuss and deal effectively with the epidemic. For this, a strategic communications plan needs to be acknowl-edged at the regional, national and community levels, where the stakeholders are clearly iden-tified and their interests are accounted, where the variety of audiences are accurately segmented, the informational and behavior change interventions are programmed and bud-geted, and so forth. Similarly, basic research will need to be commissioned to learn about the knowledge, attitudes and practices of the vulnerable populations, baselines to monitor and evaluate progress, message testing and appropriate diffusion channels will need to be selected.

On the other hand, groups with high-risk behaviors, largely identified and mapped, demand increased and focused interventions of the kind being currently tested by NGO's, with the support/experience of international donors. Public health actions (such as drug substitution, harm reduction, training CSW in negotiating techniques) *need not* be publicized, except within the IDU and CSWs groups themselves.

Concomitantly, high-level lobbying with senior politicians and parliamentarians to decriminalize high-risk behaviors, and legitimize and protect organizations working with these extremely vulnerable groups, is crucial. Attending effectively the high-risk behavior popula-tion will also provide the lead time necessary to implement a multi-sectoral approach, to contend with the next phase of the epidemic as it starts spreading to the general population.

In previous chapters, the multitude of stakeholders and their interests, as well as the institutional capacity, elements which will have an impact on project design and imple-mentation, are detailed. For the purpose of the communication activities, it can be succinctly said that, although strategic communications capacity exists in the private and academic sectors of society, it is not present in the health and educational institutions.

In order to move forward with the design of a communications strategy for the region and countries, some ideas are presented to generate discussion. These ideas will need to be expanded and modified according to the momentum of the national and regional programs, and their constituents.

Proposed Short-Term Communication Objectives

There is a three-to-five-year window of opportunity where the epidemic may be managed and possibly controlled, if effective and focused health prevention, strategic communications and harm-reduction activities take place. As support to operations, communication activi-ties can be considered at three levels: regional, national and community-based.

Regional Communications. Within the five-country region, there is a need to:

- Generate visibility among public/private decisionmakers about HIV/AIDS and its financial, social, and national security implications, while promoting political commitment and civil leadership to address the epidemic *as a development problem*.
- Position multilateral, bilateral and private donors as conveners and catalyst of best practice, in the regional fight against HIV/AIDS.

National Communications. At the country level, there is the need to create institutional capacity to:

■ Design an overarching communications strategy to support the country's HIV/AIDS programs and priorities, pursuing a multi-sectoral approach, while addressing a variety of stakeholders and their interests.

■ Raise public awareness about the alternative scenarios of the epidemic, adapting data to the peculiarities of priority audiences of each country.

■ Facilitate informed self-risk assessment and promote preventive health practices with the population at risk.

■ Foster an "enabling environment" by reducing barriers that contribute to the high incidence of the disease (denial, stigma, drug consumption, legislation that criminalizes high-risk behaviors, and so forth).

Community-based Communications. Public information and education is needed to:

■ Mobilize communities to promote participation, tapping into the existing cultural, private and faith-based organizations to secure a sustained, caring and effective outreach service.

■ Introduce behavior-change mechanisms among vulnerable populations (particularly women, youth and children).

In synthesis, communication activities are necessary at different levels. *As a region*, disclosing information about the future scenarios is vital for enabling an environment that facilitates change. At *the country level*, communication activities will motivate and give credit to the political and civil leadership, support the multi-sectoral approach, reduce the stigma and persecution of those most at risk. Strategic communications at the *community level* will solicit the mobilization of group resources, generating responses tuned to the prevailing values and beliefs, increasing sustainability and effectiveness.

Short-term Communication Activities

Regional Communications. Within a short–time perspective (two years), priority should be given to creating among political decision makers a sense of urgency to manage the *financial impacts* of HIV/AIDS (economic costs in the health sector, reduction of the productive workforce, deterioration of the investment climate, and so forth), *social costs* (reduced incentives and expectations in the vulnerable youth with its ramifications to drug consumption, sex-trade, crime, violence, social isolation, and so forth), and in terms of *national security* (diminished human and economic capacity to transform the resources of the region, increasing foreign interests to access those resources, causing immigration, political instability, and so forth).

A way to generate a sense of urgency at different levels of the population, would be to prepare and showcase the study on the possible impacts of the HIV/AIDS pandemic in the region, with a high, medium and low case scenarios. Similar to the "Russian HIV/AIDS

Modeling," this study would be presented to select high-level political authorities, members of parliament, academics and/or social critics of the five countries, in a series of meetings organized by a "Consortium" of multilateral-bilateral donors, their affiliates, and some local counterparts. At the same time, the informational event would highlight findings of other studies undertaken by the World Bank (Country Profiles), USAID (regional HIV/AIDS strategy, mapping techniques and targeted interventions in drug-demand reduction/substitution, social marketing, counseling commercial-sex workers), Global Fund (disclosure of financial resources being made available and areas of support), UNAIDS (knowledge sharing of best practices), UNICEF (educating youth), DfID and other partners.

A launching event for the modeling study would aim at bringing together Deputy Ministers, Ministers of Finance and other presidential advisors of the five Republics. The event would be linked via satellite to four other regional sites where local public officials, media, and academic representatives could participate and engage in the information-sharing opportunity.

It is crucial that in this initial event, the information to be shared centers around the financial consequences and the development impact of AIDS, as well as the benefits of early interventions involving a multi-sectoral approach. The event *should not* be a forum for the discussion of human-rights or other important social concerns.

The Global AIDS Unit of the Bank could be an important partner in the launching of this event, as they would introduce the historic perspective of the pandemic as experienced in different regions of the world, and stresses the impact of the disease in the social and economic development as well as the "investment climate" of the region (from the private sector to the donor's perspective).

From the examples stemming out of the modeling and country profiles data, as well as from the regional strategies of donors, targeted activities of their affiliates and community responses, a regional media campaign could be designed and implemented to illustrate: numbers, scenarios, development impact, vulnerable populations and most importantly, the need to stop denial.

The campaign, endorsed by the "Consortium," will secure free media time negotiated with the governments of the region, as counterparts in the process. ECA/EXT, the Global Campaigns Group of EXT, trust funds and donors could be approached to consider funding high-quality multimedia productions. Major advertising groups would be invited by the "Consortium" to collaborate, pro-bono, with their creative services. In turn, the Consortium could reciprocate by highlighting and offering international social credit and recognition to the different communication partners working in the regional approach to fight HIV/AIDS.

The collaboration and presence of the Global AIDS Unit of the Bank, could help position the institution as one of convener, and not only as a financial arm to the activities. At the same time, important initiatives may be facilitated by strong donor/funder coordination in their lobbying efforts with the Republics (increased public investments in the multi-sectoral approach, policies that decriminalize risk-behaviors, war against drug-trade, empowerment and public participation in the design and management of HIV/AIDS programs, and so forth). All of these actions could consider communication interventions in due time.

Another important asset that the Bank could mobilize is the Parliamentarian Network (PN) in the European EXT/VP, to introduce the discussion of the HIV/AIDS problem in the regional houses of representatives, focusing once again, on the financial costs for the Republics. Concomitantly, the PN could foster exchange visits of local MP's to other countries, where best practice in the civic response to AIDS can be showcased. Lastly, the Bank's Development Dialogue on Values and Ethics Unit, has collaborated with regional HIV/AIDS events, catalyzing the participation and involvement of faith-based organizations, for the committed and quality response that these groups can offer.

National Communications. As regional countries design their Health/HIV-AIDS collaborative projects, it is important to introduce and budget the communications component before the appraisal phase. This will involve TA from the Bank to the local counterparts in the preparation of a communications needs assessment, compile existing research generated by the different international and national partners, and fill the information gaps that might exist (particularly baseline information and KAP studies to understand the behaviors that need to be changed, and the activities/incentives that are likely to support those changes).

Identifying the stakeholders interests, the barriers and opportunities, and institutional capacity in the implementing organizations, constitute the initial steps towards the design of a national strategic communications plan. The plan should include other activities, like the design and testing of informational messages to specific audiences, the production of those messages in multimedia formats, and the selection and contracting of the appropriate communications channels. Monitoring and evaluation of the impact and reach of those materials, should be an activity commissioned to the intended beneficiaries.

To facilitate the adoption of a multi-sectoral approach, both for service delivery as for prevention activities, satellite distance-teaching modules have been produced by the Development Communications Unit of EXT and the World Bank Institute. These modules have trained and created institutional capacity within different ministries/service delivery organizations in Africa and South Asia. Getting public officials, NGO's and independent organizations together, sharing perspectives and alternatives, has proved invaluable to catalyze programs and empower social participation.

Similarly, the World Bank Institute has designed a distance teaching module aimed at journalists to increase the quality of reporting the epidemic, maintain the topic in the national agenda and sustain the community response. OSI/Soros Foundation and the INTERNEWS project funded by USAID, could be important partners in these activities, as they have already obtained the participation and commitment of independent broadcasting organizations, journalists and professional communicators in some Republics of Central Asia.

Following the initial regional campaign, a country-specific media campaigns would adapt the data from the modeling study to the particular circumstances of each Republic. As in the regional public information campaign, political buy-in and the contribution of the local broadcasting organizations will be sought. The costs to be incurred for the design and production of professional messages would be budgeted as part of the country programs, to be financed with national and donor resources.

In the country-based campaigns, the vulnerability of some groups needs to be highlighted (thereby promoting self-risk assessment), and stressing the importance of information and prevention. In some of the Republics, national governments have mandated that the educational curricula at the basic, middle and professional levels, educate and inform about reproductive health issues. This opportunity should be utilized to deal with the informational and cultural barriers that have an impact on the spread of the disease (denial, stigma, drug-consumption, persecution of high-risk behaviors, STD, and so forth). International NGO's contracted to work in the region have started to use this space within the school system, creating experiences that can be scaled up in the future, if resources are secured for technical expertise in curricula development, informational/educational audio-visual materials, and the training of volunteers that can extend the experience into the larger educational system. This activity and the opportunity of using the school-system as an effective information channel, is probably the most cost-effective approach in the long-term, and should be considered along with the urgent short-term interventions that are being presented.

The work undertaken by USAID financed international NGO's, such as AIDS Foundation East-West and the harm-reduction programs of OSI/Soros Foundation, will eventually need to have the political endorsement and financial support to scale up their interventions. Although these groups shy away from any type of visibility, as their approach is to slowly build trust and respect with their local counterparts (mostly the Judiciary and Police), sooner more than latter, they will require extra financial support when time comes to expand their experience to a larger portion of their beneficiary population.

Lastly, positive impacts on public awareness and change of behavior/practices will only be achieved if there is continuous availability of social products, widely distributed, of quality and at an affordable price (condoms and other physical barriers to infection). Not only do larger projects need to be aware of the importance of the social marketing efforts, but also of the vulnerability of these programs when competing activities are funded, unaware of the consequences that they create in carefully built markets (such as massive and free distribution of condoms).

Community-Based Communications. Public information will not suffice nor preclude the need to establish effective and sustainable mechanisms to reach the high risk groups, extend quality basic health services, offer counseling, testing, treatment, and accompany behavior change.

In order to increase participation, the national programs will have to tap into the credibility, of the cultural and faith-based organizations, capable of managing culturally appropriate outreach mechanisms, using peers and community volunteers to establish contact with the high-risk groups.

There are a growing number of organizations well inserted into the social fabric, some with a long-history of committed involvement, whose activities need to be funded with the necessary technical and financial resources to build-up a responsive civil society.

One way of supporting these organizations is to consider endorsing the "outreach activities" of the AIDS programs for their control and operation. The "Trust Point" centers for example, would be far more efficient and credible if managed by the communities and their representatives (including cultural and faith-based groups). They would be more likely to understand and visualize rapid research techniques, analyze the results and share them between the different stakeholders, provide informed counseling and referral services, develop informational and educational materials and events, promote the harm-reduction and social marketing interventions, serve as sentinel points and advocate for the needs of the vulnerable and infected.

These community organizations will have to be invested with the mandate needed to undertake their difficult activity. They also need to be provided with public visibility, so that the beneficiaries know about their locations and services. It would be useful to consider in the design of national programs the inclusion of some pilot projects where the community response is accounted, supported and empowered.

Bank communication and participation activities. In addition to activities indicated above to be carried out by Governments with Bank assistance in some cases, the Bank will engage in the following specific communication and participation activities:

- The Central Asia HIV/AIDS and TB Country Profiles were translated, discussed with stakeholders, and distributed in the region and among international partner organizations.
- This study has also been translated, discussed with stakeholders, and will be distributed in the region and among international partner organizations.
- Stakeholder workshops have been organized to learn more about clients' demand for TB and HIV/AIDS activities, and build consensus on the Bank's role in this area.
- The Bank has been assisting regional Governments identifying additional funding for capacity building.
- The Bank will carry out learning activities through GDLN.

Table 23. Communication Plan

Level	Objective	Priority Audience	Activity	Intervention	Time to Execute	Preliminary Costs
Regional Level Communication Activities	Acknowledgement of financial, social and national security costs associated with HIV/AIDS.	Political decision makers, parliament, academics, and social critics.	Diffusion of Central Asian modeling study and other donors studies.	Main launching event and satellite links with 4 participating sites in the rest of the CA countries.	5 months from project start	$15,000
	Social awareness of the associated costs of HIV/AIDS to the region.	Educated population of the 5 Republics, private sector, and vulnerable groups	Adapt information stemming from modeling study and diffuse it though technical channels	Produce and distribute regional campaigns in electronic and print media in 5 republics.	8 months from project start	$90,000 for production costs
National Level Communication Activities	Develop national strategic communications plans	Counterparts and beneficiaries	Needs assessment, compile existing research (baseline and KAP studies) stakeholder and institutional analysis, design and testing of messages, select communication channels, monitoring and evaluation.	TA from Bank staff and consultants to the counterpart agencies of five CA countries.	8 months from project start	$60,000
	Facilitate adoption of a multi-sectoral approach to service delivery and preventive actions	Segmented audiences and beneficiaries	Transmit and train selected ministries in 5 countries, through distance teaching tools.	Enroll trainees and broadcast distance-teaching modules.	12 months from project start	$80,000
	Independent press reporting the epidemic with quality and accuracy	Media professionals.	Training courses for journalists.	One training course for each country.	15 months from project start	$50,000

Social awareness about the epidemic and how it might affect vulnerable groups.	Women, youth	Adapt modeling study to specific conditions of each country's vulnerable population.	Produce and diffuse media campaigns in the 5 Republics.	12 months from project start	$110,000
Use the educational system to mainstream reproductive health and HIV/AIDS prevention.	Young audiences	Develop educational AV materials around denial, stigma and discrimination, drug consumption, preventive measures.	Design and produce AV materials, train volunteers and distribute the educational packages.	15 months from project start	$30,000
Harm reduction and drug-substitution	High risk behavior groups	Focused activities related to counseling, needle exchange, and other harm-reduction interventions.	Lobby decision makers for continued support to high-risk behavior interventions.	Ongoing	
Condom distribution and social marketing of physical barriers.	High-risk and vulnerable groups	Distribution of prevention products in the "mapped" high-risk areas and eventually in large distribution networks.	Social marketing	Ongoing	
Community Level Communication Activities Empower communities to endorse the "social vaccine"	Grass-root activists and leaders	Empower community groups for outreach services, and provide social credit for their services.	Funding and training of grass-root organizations in counseling, testing, referring and social marketing activities.	20 months from project start	$110,000

Bibliography

Adeyi, O., and others. 2003. *Averting AIDS Crises in Eastern Europe and Central Asia—A Regional Support Strategy.* Washington, D.C.: The World Bank.

AIDS Center. 2004. "Public Opinion Research on Awareness, Attitudes and Practices regarding HIV/AIDS in Kazakhstan." Survey was carried out in the context of the GFATM Grant Application.

Arnstein, S. 1969. "A Ladder of Citizen Participation." *Journal of American Institute of Planners* 35(4):216–224.

Asian Development Bank. 2001. "Kazakhstan Country Report." Online.

Bardach, E. 1998. *Getting Agencies to Work Together.* Washington, D.C.: Brookings Institution Press.

Basmakova and others. 2003. *AIDS in Kyrgyz Republic: five years resistance.*

Bernard, D., and others. 2001. *Societies in Transition: A Situational Analysis of the Status of Children and Women in the Central Asian Republics and Kazakhstan.* Almaty: UNICEF.

Brown, T., B. Franklin, J. McNeil, and S. Mills. 2001. *Effective Prevention Strategies in Low HIV Prevalence Settings.* Arlington: Family Health International.

Burns, M., and H. Morgan. 2001. "Breaking Through Barriers of Fear, Myth and Jargon: How we teach HIV transmission at AIDSLINE." Sixth International Congress on AIDS in Asia and the Pacific, Melbourne, October 5–10.

Cercone, J., and others. Forthcoming. *Kazakhstan TB and HIV/AIDS Program Review.* The Government of Kazakhstan and the World Bank.

Coates, T.J. 2000. "Efficacy of Voluntary HIV–1 Counseling and Testing in Individuals and Couples in Kenya, Tanzania, and Trinidad: A Randomised Trial." *Lancet* 356(9224): 103–112.

Dallabetta, G., and S. Gavrilin. 2001. "Assessment of the HIV situation in selected sites in Kyrgyz Republic, Uzbekistan and Kazakhstan." IMPACT/Family Health International Report prepared for USAID/Regional Mission to Central Asia. Available at http://www.dec.org/pdf_docs/PNACP295.pdf

Dehne, K.L., and Y. Kobyscha. 2000. "The HIV epidemic in Central and Eastern Europe: Update 2000." A Report to a Second Strategy Meeting to Better Coordinate Regional Support to National Responses to HIV/AIDS in Central and Eastern Europe, December 4–5, Copenhagen.

Defty, H. 2002. *Infrequent Injection Drug Users: Research and interventions with young people at risk of HIV, with special focus on CEE/CIS and the Baltics.* Vienna: UNAIDS.

Des Jarlais, D. 2000. "HIV Incidence Among Injection Drug Users in New York City, 1992–1997: Evidence for a Declining Epidemic." *American Journal of Public Health* 90(3):352–359.

Des Jarlais, D., and S.R. Friedman. 1994. "AIDS and the Use of Injected Drugs." *Scientific American* (February):82–88.

Des Jarlais, D., and others. 1996. "HIV Incidence among Injecting Drug Users in New York City Syringe-Exchange Programs." *Lancet* 348(9033):987–991.

DFID. 2004. "Concept Paper for a grant for prevention of HIV/AIDS in Central Asia."

Drucker, E. 1995. "Harm Reduction: A Public Health Strategy." *Current Issues in Public Health* 1:64–70.

European Observatory on Health Care Systems. 2000. *Health Care Systems in Transition: Kyrgyz Republic.* Copenhagen: WHO.

Express. 1998. *Situation analysis of the prevalence of IDU and the possibility of an outbreak of an HIV epidemic.*

Felzer, S. 2004. *Public Opinion research on HIV/AIDS in the Kyrgyz Republic and Albania.* Washington, D.C.: The World Bank.

Global HIV Prevention Working Group. 2002. "Global Mobilization for HIV Prevention: A Blueprint for Action." Available at http://www.kff.org/hivaids/2002–07-index.cfm

Godinho, J., T. Novotny, H. Tadesse, and A. Vinokur. 2004. *HIV/AIDS and Tuberculosis in Central Asia: Country Profiles.* World Bank Working Paper No. 20. Washington, D.C.: The World Bank.

Godinho, and others. Forthcoming. *HIV/AIDS in the Western Balkans.* Washington, D.C.: The World Bank.

Godinho J., J. Veen, M. Dara, J. Cercone, and J. Pacheco. Forthcoming. *Stopping TB in Central Asia.* Washington, D.C.: The World Bank.

Gotsadze, G. 2003. *HIV/AIDS Country Report: Kazakhstan.* 2004. "Social and Institutional Assessment." Central Asia HIV/AIDS Control Project PreparationDocument.

Gotsadze, T., Chawla M, and Chkatarashvili K. 2004. *HIV/AIDS in Georgia: Addressing the Crisis.* World Bank Working Paper No. 23. Washington, D.C.: The World Bank.

Grosskurth, H., and others. 1995. "Impact of improved treatment of sexually transmitted diseases on HIV infection in rural Tanzania." *Lancet* 346:530–536.

Grund, J.P. 2001. "A Candle Lit from Both Sides: The Epidemic of HIV Infection in Central and Eastern Europe." In K. McElrath, ed., *HIV and AIDS: A Global View.* Westport, Conn.: Greenwood Press.

Hamers, F.F., and A.M. Downs. 2003. "HIV in Central and Eastern Europe." *Lancet*, 361(9362):1035–104.

Hanenberg, R.S., D.C. Sokal., W. Rojanapithayakorn., and P. Kunasol. 1994. "Impact of Thailand's HIV-control program as indicated by the decline of sexually transmitted diseases." *Lancet* 344 (8917):243–245.

Human Rights Watch. 2003. "Fanning the Flames: How Human Rights Abuses are Fueling the AIDS Epidemic in Kazakhstan." http://www.hrw.org/reports/2003/kazak0603/kazak0603.pdf

Hurley, S., and others. 1997. "Effectiveness of needle-exchange programs for prevention of HIV infection." *Lancet* 349(9068):1797–1800.

Joshua, L. 2003. "World Bank Social Insurance Technical Assistance Project [SITAP]." Pensions Workshop, Banja Luka, July 7–8. Based on literature addressing participatory approaches including Arnstein (1979) and Nazurov, Rose, and Shelley (2000).

Kazakh CCM. 2002. "Promotion of and support to safer behavior choices among target population groups (injecting drug users, commercial sex workers, youth); provision of care and support to people with HIV/AIDS." GFATM Grant Application, Round 2. Astana. Available at http://www.theglobalfund.org/en/about/publications/

Kroll, C. 2002. "Assistance to Country Responses on HIV/AIDS Associated with Injecting Drug Use by the UN and Other Agencies." Report for the Interagency Task Team on Injecting Drug Use, July 29–30, Geneva.

Kyrgyz Republic. 2001. "The State Program on Prevention of AIDS, Infections Transmitted via Sexual and Injecting Ways for 2001–2005." Bishkek. Available at http://www.undp.kg/english/pubs10.phtml

Kyrgyz Republic CCM. 2002. "Development of preventive programmes on HIV/AIDS, Tuberculosis and Malaria aimed at reduction of social and economic consequences of their spread." GFATM Grant Application, Round 2. Bishkek. Available at http://www.theglobalfund.org/en/about/publications/

Kyrgyz Republic and UNDP. 2003. *Common Country Assessment.* Bishkek: UNDP.

Kulis, M., and M. Chawla. 2004. *Truck Drivers and Casual Sex: An Inquiry into the Potential Spread of HIV/AIDS in the Baltic Region.* World Bank Working Paper No. 37. Washington, D.C.: The World Bank.

Kumaranayake, L., C. Watts, P. Vickerman, and D. Walker. 2003. "Cost-effectiveness of HIV preventive measures among injecting drug users." *UNAIDS Best Practice Digest.*

Kumpl, F., and S. Franke. 2002. "Needs Assessment on Drug Abuse in the Central Asian Countries." Project No. AD/RER/01/F08, Working Paper. Vienna.

Lubin, N., A. Klaits, and I. Barsegian. 2002. *Narcotics Interdiction in Afghanistan and Central Asia: Challenges for International Assistance.* A Report to the Open Society Institute's Central Eurasia Project and Network of Women's Programs. New York, Open Society Institute.

Miller, D., and others. 2004. *Surveillance Systems in Eastern Europe and Central Asia.* Washington, D.C.: The World Bank

Mugrditchian, D. 2001. Conference on the Prevention of HIV/AIDS and Sexually Transmitted Infections in Central Asia. Almaty.

Needle, R. and others. 1998. "HIV prevention with drug-using populations—current status and future prospects: introduction and overview." *Public Health Reports* 113(Suppl 1):4–30.

Novotny, T., D. Haazen, and O. Adeyi. 2003. *HIV/AIDS in Southeastern Europe: Case Studies from Bulgaria, Croatia, and Romania.* World Bank Working Paper No. 4. Washington, D.C.: The World Bank.

Oostvogels. 1999. "Overview of Outreach work among CSWs and their clients in Kyrgyz Republic, October 1998–April 1999." UNAIDS/WHO Consultant Report.

Open Society Institute. 2002. *Sex Worker Harm Reduction Initiative Mid-Year Report: A Guide to Contacts and Services in Central and Eastern Europe and the Former Soviet Union.* International Harm Reduction Development Program. Budapest.

———. 2003. *DDRP Consolidated Assessment.*

———. 2004. *Breaking Down Barriers: Lessons on Providing HIV Treatment to Injection Drug Users.* International Harm Reduction Development Program. New York. Available at http://www.soros.org/initiatives/ihrd/articles_publications/publications/arv_idus _20040715

Peddro. 2001. "Drug Abuse and AIDS—Stemming the Epidemic." Newsletter, Special Issues. UNESCO, the European Commission and Onusida. December.

Pokrovsky, V. 1996. *Epidemiology and Prevention of HIV Infection and AIDS*. Moscow: Meditsina Publ.

Population Services International. 2001. *Social Marketing Assessment for HIV/STI Prevention in the Central Asian Republics of Kazakhstan, Kyrgyz Republic and Uzbekistan*.

Power, R., and N. Nozhkina. 2002. "The value of process evaluation in sustaining HIV harm reduction in the Russian Federation." *AIDS* 16(2):303–304.

Rahmonov, E. 2000. Statement About National Program on Prevention and Control Against Human Immunodeficiency Virus, Acquired Immunodeficiency Syndrome and Sexually Transmitted Diseases in Republic of Tajikistan for the Period Till the Year 2007.

Renton, A., D. Gzirishvili, G. Gotsadze, and J. Godinho. Forthcoming. *Epidemics and Drivers: Regional Challenge, Regional Response*. London: Imperial College/DFID/The World Bank.

River, M.J., G. Gotsadze, A. Amato-Gauci, and N. Kerimi. 2003. "Stakeholders Analysis." Central Asia HIV/AIDS Control Project Preparation Document.

Ruhl, C., V. Vinogradov, V. Pokrovsky, and N. Ladnaya. 2003. *The Economic Consequences of HIV in Russia*. Moscow: The World Bank.

Saidel, T.J., and others. 2003. "Potential impact of HIV among IDUs on heterosexual -transmission in Asian settings: scenarios from the Asian Epidemic Model." *The International Journal of Drug Policy* 14:63–74.

Soderland, N., J. Lavis, J. Broomberg, and A. Mills. 1993. "The costs of HIV prevention strategies in developing countries." *Bulletin of the World Health Organization* 71:595–604.

Stachowiak, J., and C. Beyrer. 2002. "HIV follows heroin trafficking routes." Presentation at the Conference Health Security in Central Asia: Drug Use, HIV, and AIDS, Dushanbe, October 14–16. Available at http://www.eurasianet.org/health.security/presentations/hiv_trafficking.shtml

Stimson, G.V., L.J. Alldritt, and K.A. Dolan. 1998. *Injecting Equipment Exchange Schemes: Final Report*. London: University of London/Goldsmiths College/Monitoring Research Group.

Tajik CCM. 2002. Support to the Strategic Plan of the National Response to the HIV/AIDS epidemics in prevention activities among IDU, SW and youth and envisaging blood safety in Tajjikistan. GFATM Grant Application. Round 1. Dushanbe. Available at http://www.theglobalfund.org/en/about/publications/

———. 2004. "Reducing the Burden of HIV/AIDS in Tajikistan." GFATM Grant Application, Round 4. Dushanbe. Available at http://www.theglobalfund.org/search/docs/4TAJH_821_0_full.pdf

Thomas, R.M. 1996. *Assessment of Commercial Sex Scene in Almaty, Kazakhstan*. Almaty: UNAIDS.

Tokayev, K. 2001. "On the Approval of the Program to Counteract the AIDS Epidemic in the Republic of Kazakhstan for 2001–2005." Resolution of the Government of the Republic of Kazakhstan. Almaty.

Turkmenbashi, S. 2001. "Law of Turkmenistan on Prophylactics of Disease, Casused by Human Immunodeficiency Virus (HIV-Infection)." Ashgabat.

UN. 2001. *The Millennium Development Goals*. New York.

UNAIDS. 2001. *HIV Prevention Needs and Successes: a tale of three countries*.

———. 2001a. "AIDS Epidemic Update." Available at http://www.who.int/hiv/pub/epidemiology/epi2001/en/

————. 2001b. *UNAIDS Assisted Response to HIV/AIDS, STIs, and Drug Abuse in Central Asian Countries (Kazakhstan, Kyrgyz Republic, Tajikistan, Turkmenistan, and Uzbekistan),* 1996–2000. Almaty.

————. 2002. "AIDS Epidemic Update." Available at http://www.who.int/hiv/pub/epidemiology/epi2002/en/

————. 2002a. *UNAIDS Task Force on HIV Prevention Among Injecting Drug Users in Eastern Europe and the Newly Independent States.* Facts Sheet. Vienna.

————. 2002b. *UN Interagency Group for Young People's Health Development and Protection in Europe and Central Asia (IAG).* Geneva: UNICEF.

————. 2002c. *Rapid Assessment Report.*

————. 2003. "AIDS Epidemic Update." Available at http://www.unaids.org/Unaids/EN/Resources/Publications/

————. 2004. "AIDS Epidemic Update." Available at http://www.unaids.org/wad2004/report.html

UNAIDS and The World Bank. 2003. *Funding requirements for the response to HIV/AIDS in ECA.*

UNDP. 2002. *Non-Governmental Organizations of Kazakhstan: Past, Present, Future.* Almaty.

————. 2003. *Human Development Report.* New York.

UNFPA. 2001. *Peer-led Sexuality Education—Results of the Knowledge, Attitudes, Practices, and Behaviour (KAPB) Survey.* IPPF EN Field Office for Central Asia, Almaty.

UNICEF. 2001. *A Developmental and Emergency Response to HIV/AIDS Among Young Drug Users in the CEE/CIS/Baltics Region—A Review Paper.* UNICEF Regional Office for CEE/CID/Baltics. Geneva.

————. 2002. "Consultation with Partners to Assist UNICEF in Clarifying its Role and Plans for IDU-Related Programming on Young People and HIV/AIDS in the CEE/CIS and the Baltic States." April 16 Draft Report. Geneva.

————. 2003. *Rapid Assessment and Response to HIV/AIDS Among Especially Vulnerable Young People in Tajikistan.* Dushanbe.

UNODC. 2001. *Global Illicit Drug Trends.* Available at http://www.unodc.org/pdf/report_2001–06–26_1/report_2001–06–26_1.pdf

————. 2002. *Illicit Drugs Situation in the Regions Neighbouring Afghanistan and the Response of ODC.* Available at http://www.unodc.org/pdf/afg/afg_drug-situation_2002–11–01_1.pdf

————. 2003. *Audit on the Number of Injecting Drug Users in Central Eastern Europe and Central Asia.*

USAID.2002. "USAID's Strategy on HIV/AIDS Prevention in Central Asia 2002–2004." Available at http://www.usaid.gov/our_work/global_health/aids/Countries/eande/caregion.html

————. 2003. "Kazakhstan Country Summary from the fiscal year 2003."

————. 2003a. *Drug prevention and HIV/AIDS epidemic in Central Asia.*

————. 2003c. *HIV/AIDS Epidemic in Central Asia—Projections.*

————. 2003d. *PLACE Methodology.* MEASURE Evaluation Project, University of North Carolina. Available at http://www.usaid.gov/locations/europe_eurasia/car/hiv_aids/measure.htm

USAID and Central Asia Republics (CAR) Centers for Disease Control and Prevention (CDC). 2003. "Program for Infectious Disease Control."

USAID and the Synergy Project. 2002. *What Happened in Uganda? Declining HIV Prevalence, Behavior Change, and the National Response*. Project Lessons Learned Case Study. Washington, D.C.: The Synergy Project.

U.S. Centers for Disease Control and Prevention (CDC). 2003a. "Advancing HIV Prevention: New Strategies for a Changing Epidemic—United States, 2003." *Morbidity and Mortality Weekly Report* 52(15):329–332.

———. 2003b. "Rapid increase in HIV rates—Orel Oblast, Russian Federation, 1999–2001." *Morbidity and Mortality Weekly Report* 52(28):656–660.

Uzbek CCM. 2003. "Scaling up the Response to HIV/AIDS: A Focus on Vulnerable Populations." GFATM Grant Application, Round 3. Tashkent. Available at http://www.theglobalfund.org/en/about/publications/

Uzbekistan, Republic of. 2002. "Strategic Program on Counteraction to HIV/AIDS Epidemic Expansion in the Republic of Uzbekistan." Cabinet of Ministers of the Republic of Uzbekistan. Tashkent.

Van Empelen, P., and others. 2003. "Effective methods to change sex-risk among drug users: a review of psychosocial interventions." *Social Science Medicine* 57(9):1593–608.

WHO and UNAIDS. 2000. *Guidelines for Second Generation HIV Surveillance for HIV: The Next Decade*. Geneva: World Health Organization (WHO/CDS/EDC/2000.05).

WHO, UNFPA, and UNICEF. 1997. *Action for Adolescent Health: Towards a Common Agenda*. Geneva.

WHO Europe. 2002. "Task Force for STI Prevention and Care in Eastern Europe and Central Asia." Presented at the South Eastern Europe Conference on HIV/AIDS: Implementing the Global Declaration of Commitment on HIV/AIDS, June 6–8, Bucharest, Romania.

WHO Information Centre on Health for CAR. 2003. *Drugs in Central Asia*.

World Bank. 2003. *Averting AIDS Crisis in Eastern Europe and Central Asia—A regional Support Strategy*. Washington, D.C.

———. 2003a. *Health in Europe and Central Asia: Business Plan for 2003–2007*. Washington, D.C.

———. 2004. "Uzbek Health II Project Appraisal Document." Washington, D.C.

———. 2004a. *Kyrgyz Republic Public Expenditure Review*. Volume 1. Washington, D.C.

———. Undated. "Central Asia AIDS Control Project Appraisal Document." Washington, D.C.

Zhusupov, B. 2000. "Women, Youth and HIV/AIDS in Kazakhstan." Expert Group Meeting on the HIV/AIDS Pandemic and its Gender Implications, November 13–17, Windhoek. Available at http://www.un.org/womenwatch/daw/csw/hivaids/Zhusupov.html